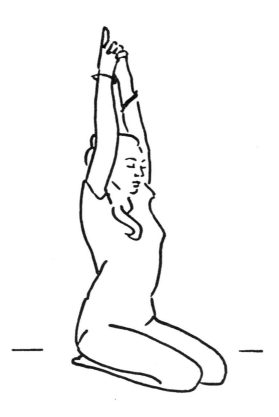

YOGA FOR HEALTH AND HEALING

From the Teachings of
Yogi Bhajan, Ph.D.

Compiled by Alice Clagett and Elandra Kirsten Meredith
Cover Design by Award-Winning Graphic Designer Robin Weisz
Photographed by Ardas Kaur Khalsa
Edited by Susanna Contini Hennink
Posed by Elandra Kirsten Meredith
Cover Pose by Heather Luna Keasbey

Yoga for Health and Healing

ISBN 0-940992-01-9 ❖ $14.95 ❖ Trade Paperback
SAN 219-6719

Revised in 1994
Second Printing in 1995
Printed in the United States of America

For additional copies of this book, write to:

Alice B. Clagett
P.O. Box 3142
Santa Monica, CA 90408

Phone: (310) 393-8167
Fax: (310) 393-8167

Also distributed by A & S, Ancient Healing Ways, Baker & Taylor, Bookpeople, Golden Lee, Golden Temple Enterprises, Ingram, and New Leaf.

5/95

to Deke

ACKNOWLEDGMENTS

Yoga for Health and Healing would never have been possible without the help of a number of dedicated people who have compiled Yogi Bhajan's teaching on the topic. Special thanks are due M.S.S. Gurucharan Singh Khalsa for much of the information in Chapters 1 and 2, and for the section on "Sleep" in Appendix A.

The book as a whole is based on the teachings of Yogi Bhajan, always a source of wisdom and inspiration.

NOTE

This book is a reference work. It is not intended to be a replacement for competent medical care. The directions stated are not intended as a prescription for any mental or physical ailments, nor does the information claim treatment or cure for any problems.

FOREWORD

When Yogi Bhajan, master of white tantric yoga and kundalini yoga, arrived in the United States in January of 1969, he created an uproar among his Indian friends and acquaintances by introducing to his yoga students hundreds of practical kundalini yoga techniques for healing and uplifting body, mind, and spirit.

These techniques, which incorporate the major features of all other yogas except tantric yoga, are streamlined and efficient. They are said to achieve in a year what it takes 12 years of hatha yoga to achieve.

This manual contains excellent, fast-acting kundalini yoga techniques and meditations for self-healing. If you have never practiced kundalini yoga before, read Chapter 1 to gain an understanding of yogic theory and Chapter 2 for an introduction to the basics of yogic practice. (For a self-healing experience that defies description, try practicing "Sat Kriya," found at the end of Chapter 1, 31 minutes a day for 40 days.)

The remaining chapters will give you the necessary tools to maintain a healthy body (Chapter 3), to help correct specific physical and mental problems (Chapter 4), and to develop your ability to heal others (Chapter 5).

It's important to keep in mind the fact that yoga is only one aspect of self-healing. Particularly for severe problems, be sure to consult your health care specialist. Since lifestyle has a significant influence on health, the yogic concept of a healthful lifestyle is described in Appendix A.

If you would like to practice kundalini yoga in a group, you can call one of the Kundalini Yoga Teaching Centers listed in Appendix B and ask for information on classes near you.

We hope that all our readers will be blessed with good health and a long, happy life!

CONTENTS

1. YOGA AS A TOOL FOR SELF-HEALING

Yoga has long been thought of as a form of preventive health care—one does hatha yoga, for instance, to maintain physical vitality and flexibility. But the advent of kundalini yoga, with its fast-acting, specific applications to a wide range of health problems, places the science of yoga in the cadres of such self-help techniques as acupressure, therapeutic massage, herbal medicine, and healthful diet as an active means of improving health.

The theory of yoga incorporates many principles that are currently beyond the understanding of science. Like acupressure and acupuncture, yoga works with human energies so subtle that modern science has not the instruments to measure them, much less the ability to verify their existence. These energies are not so subtle that they cannot be experienced by you and me, however. That is how they were discovered in the first place: through the conscious experience of those who made their minds and bodies still enough to tune in to these subtle forces. This chapter describes aspects of yogic science as yet unexplored by modern science. Wherever possible, we suggest experiments that you can do so as to experience their application firsthand.

Ten Bodies

Much of yogic science deals with aspects of the physical body already known to modern science.[1] It offers ways to cleanse the circula-

----
[1]For sets of exercises dealing with maintenance of basic body systems, see the **Sadhana Guidelines** and **Maintenance Yoga** (Appendix C).

tory system and relieve it of stress, to improve the efficiency and correct malfunctions of the digestive tract, to flush out the lymphatic system, to bolster the immune system, to tune and balance the nervous system, to stretch and tone the muscles, and to revitalize the reproductive system. A large portion of yogic science deals specifically with regulating the function of the endocrine system—the dozens of hormones that, along with the nervous system, act as an interface between you and your environment. For reasons peculiar to the evolution of that science, to be discussed later in this chapter, certain glands, such as the pituitary and pineal, receive special emphasis.

But more than dealing with the physical body, and more than dealing with the triad of mind–body–spirit, yogic science deals with a complex, subtle skein of energies that mold us as human beings. It actually deals with 10 "bodies" or energy states: the physical, the spiritual, three kinds of mental (positive, negative, and neutral), the **arcline** and auric body (both electromagnetic), and the subtle, pranic, and radiant bodies. The relationship of these "bodies," both to themselves and to one another, is governed by the flow of several types of energy.

The Electric Force

The electric force is responsible for message carrying and proper functioning of the brain control center in the physical body. It also helps the arteries and veins carry the circulation of the blood throughout the body. It is responsible for all activities of the nerves, thoughts, and

1

Exercises to Strengthen

Do these exercises after taking a cold shower. Do them sitting on a sheepskin or wool blanket placed over a white sheet. The sheepskin will insulate the electrical charge in your spine and the white sheet will amplify the flow of your magnetic field.

1. After a cold shower, sit on your heels, joining your palms together over your head, arms hugging ears. Stretch the arms up (a) and begin **Sat Kriya** (see this chapter, "Sat Kriya to Raise the Kundalini"), pulling up and in strongly on the anus, sex organs and navel (**root lock**) as you say **SAT** ("truth"; *a* as in "bus"). This will increase your "voltage."

2. Sit in a comfortable cross-legged position with a straight spine (**easy pose**). Blocking the left nostril with your left thumb, begin long, deep breathing through your right nostril (b). With each inhale, mentally chant SAT; with each exhale mentally chant **NAAM** ("name"; *aa* as in "far").

3. Sitting in easy pose, hold your hands against the back of your neck (c) in **venus lock** (Chapter 2). Inhale deeply. Exhale deeply as you bend forward, touching your forehead to the floor (d). Then come up and lean back to 60° from the horizon, mentally chanting SAT NAAM (e). *Repeat this three-fold movement for 1-3 min.*

4. Sitting in easy pose with hands on knees, thumb and forefinger touching (**gyan mudra**), *meditate for 1-3 minutes* (f). Breath is normal.

5. Lie down on your back with your arms stretched out behind you, arms hugging ears (g). Inhale, sit up, and touch your toes (h), keeping the spine straight. Curl back down. This releases pressure on the back and adjusts the electric force.

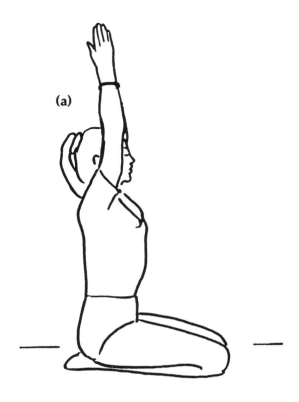

(a)

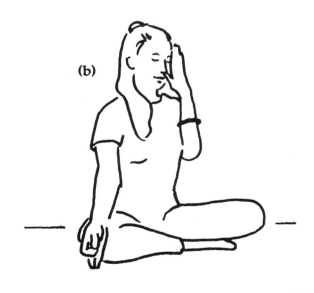

(b)

the Electric Force

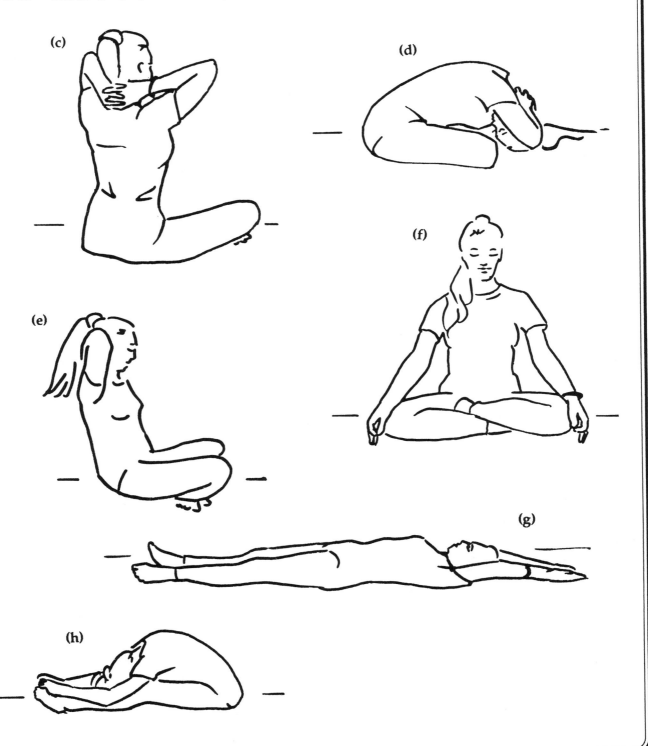

(c)

(d)

(f)

(e)

(g)

(h)

3

senses. It is self-generated. One of the functions of the hair is to protect this system. How long your hair grows when left in its natural state depends on the needs of your electric force.

In this system energy is supplied by way of the spine to the peripheral nervous system and to the blood vessels. When the voltage in a person is weak, his outlook is negative and his projection as an individual is weak.

The Magnetic Field

The magnetic field is said to rebuild the body, make a person attractive, and draw success to one's endeavors. The magnetic field is responsible for keeping the whole body together and for the functioning of the muscular system. It controls a person's strength.

The magnetic field surrounds the body in the same way the earth's magnetic field en-velops our planet. It adjusts itself every 2 1/2 hours during daylight hours. During sleep it forms a different kind of field which is particularly sensitive to disturbances. That's why it's very important not to wake from a deep sleep quickly. People who leap out of bed can do damage to their magnetic field, weakening both their personality and their muscle strength. (As a precaution, do the wake-up exercises indicated in Appendix A in the section on "Sleep" before getting up.) The magnetic field also affects our emotions and communications. It takes balanced nerves and a strong magnetic field to maintain happiness. The best way to strengthen the magnetic field is to meditate on one's breath every morning.

As the magnetic field gets stronger, you will find that you relate to emotions differently. You can choose to relate to someone or disconnect from their influence. When your radiance is

Exercises to Strengthen the Magnetic Field

1. Sit in easy pose, arms straight out from the sides, palms down. Keeping the arms straight, move them in a backwards circular motion (a). *Continue for 1 min.*

2. Still sitting in easy pose, with upper arms out to the sides and parallel to the floor, touch fingertips to shoulders (b). Inhale deeply and hold the breath in as long as you can. Exhale, relax, and feel the renewed energy circulating.*

---

*For other exercises for the magnetic field, see **Sadhana Guidelines** (Appendix C).

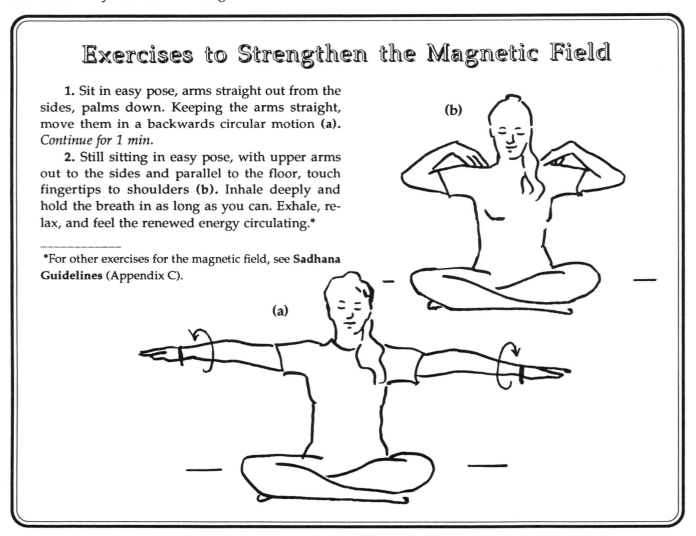

(b)

(a)

Some Straight Spine Positions

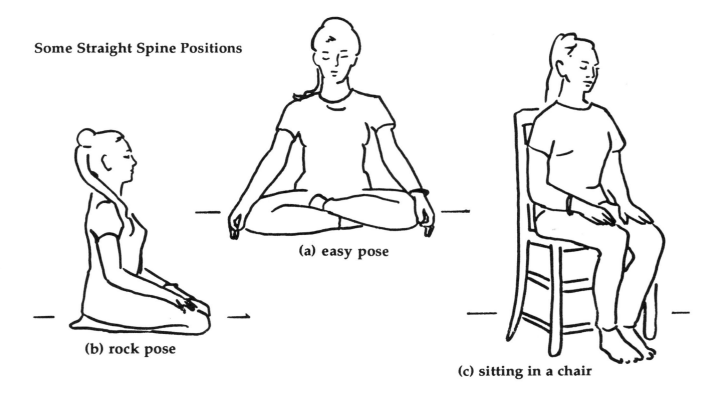

(a) easy pose

(b) rock pose

(c) sitting in a chair

strong and you direct it to someone, they will want to talk to you and be around you in spite of great differences or pains. You will find that the magnetic fields of those around you harmonize with your own—in other words, the environment will operate in tune with you. In spiritual language, they say that when a man projects God's light, all darkness flees. Wherever he goes, light, beauty, bounty and fulfillment surround him.

The Life Force

The life force comes through the breath and is, mainly, the energy on which one depends for life. It enters through the nostrils as one breathes, activating the channels of the **ida** and **pingala,** which are thought to correspond either to the sympathetic ganglia of the autonomic nervous system or to the urinary bladder meridians of acupressure. These channels draw the life force energy through the body, distributing it finally to every cell. The ida is controlled by breath through the left nostril and the pingala by breath through the right. They are represented symbolically by the energy of the moon and the sun, respectively. It is through their combined energy that the spark of life is ignited: without it, there is no life. The life force has the potential to become the kundalini energy, pervading our being with heightened energy and radiance. While it is largely brought into the body on the breath, it can also come through food and through touch.

The life force is responsible for controlling the temperature of the body, for the circulation and heartbeat, and for the purification of the blood through the lungs. The heart and diaphragm, the two organs responsible for the inflex and reflex of the lungs, are worked by the life force. When the life force touches the receiving center in the nostrils, it goes directly through the special channels along the spine. From there it passes to the heart and diaphragm muscles to make them function smoothly.

If you can sit with a straight spine (chin tucked in, chest out) for 31 min **(a,b,c),** you can increase the flow of the life force in all parts of your body. Breathing should be long and deep.

5

This exercise, which is the basic meditation pose, is best done after bathing. This practice will give one longer life, control of the mind, control of the emotions, and well-balanced behavior. It will soothe the nervous system and remove irritation, creating a soft mood that will make one feel pleasant. He will find he has a softer tone and will be magnetic to others. People will like him; he will be shored against negative and dark forces. It also makes a person openhearted, truthful, and loving. He feels everyone to be the same, and loses the distinctions by which he discriminates against others. He sees everyone else as part of the same force. If this force can be created and controlled, a person can become so powerful that he can change the destiny of others. He learns to project his force to the weak force of others, strengthening their magnetic field, cutting off negative actions against them, and relieving them of their bad luck and misfortune.

Life Force Exercise

Sit in easy pose, arms straight out in front, parallel to the ground, palms facing each other. Inhale completely with hands open (a). Then make tight fists and exhale (b), at the same time pulling up and in on the rectum, sex organs, and navel point (root lock). *Continue for 3 min.*

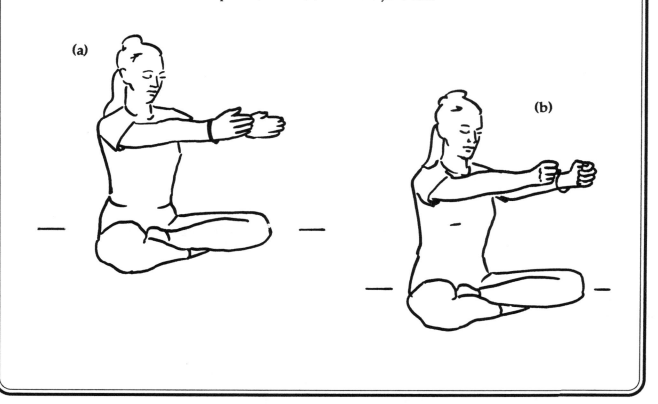

(a)

(b)

Chakras

There are eight **chakras** in the physical body: the first seven are life force centers along the spine and along the head; the last is the **aura** (outer magnetic field), which encompasses all the chakras. These chakras are points of energy transformation from the more subtle bodies of a human being to the physical body. While they are decidedly nonphysical in nature, they do, nonetheless, exist. Scientists have identified what they call an "X" force that corresponds to the chakras and to the life force, but have not yet devised a means of measuring it. The chakras are the answer to 17th century philosopher Rene Descartes' question, "How do the physical and the spiritual relate?" They do so by means of "socializing" areas known as chakras.

The name chakra, or "wheel," derives from the shape of these nerve centers. They project away from the area of the spinal column in the shape of a hub with spokes, or like a flower with petals. Different societies give different symbolic interpretations of the shape and image of each chakra. In each, their function and capacity is largely the same.

Each chakra, and the energy funneled through it, has a physical and psychological relationship to our lives. Physically, they relate to different glands and nerve complexes. Psychologically, they reflect and direct emotions and feelings of consciousness related to each specific center. These centers are archetypes for universal experiences of consciousness. They begin with the basest of elements and progress to elements normally unknown to humanity.

The first, or **root chakra,** corresponds to the earth element. It is animal function in its most necessary and most common form—elimination and survival. The **second chakra,** located roughly in the center of the pelvis, is water. It deals with sexuality and procreation. The **third chakra,** at the navel point, is fire. It corresponds to power, and can work for good or evil, though in most of us it aspires no higher than greed. It can, however, be a very high cen-

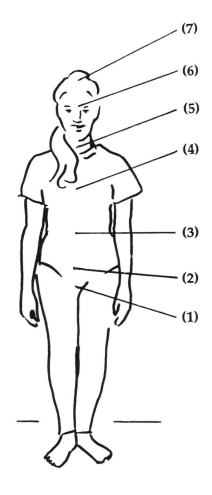

ter: it is the center from which many masters of the martial arts have drawn their awareness.

The **fourth chakra,** at the heart, is related to the air element. (As you can see, the elements are becoming progressively more subtle and elevated.) The heart chakra opens up in a person the ability to serve, to understand, and to love: to love not personalities in a person but qualities—and to assist the expansion of those qualities. Next, the **throat chakra:** the element ether, knowledge. Not just facts, but the truth: A person whose throat chakra is well developed has the power, no matter how poorly he speaks, to move people with his voice. The **sixth chakra,** at the pituitary gland, is so subtle that the English language does not have a word for it. In Sanskrit, it is called "manas." Think of

7

it as the light energy of the mind: that which illuminates. For the **seventh chakra,** at the pineal gland, the element is God. Last is the **aura** or **circumvent force,** which blends the energies and elements of all the chakras into the total human being.

Knowing these facts about the chakras is not important to their function, any more than knowing how the eye works is needed to see.

But it may help in directing the energy of your meditations and in understanding your motivations as you are influenced by different centers at different times. For instance, you may wish to take note of your state of mind right now, then do the "Meditation to Open the Heart Chakra" (see illustration). After you've finished, compare states of mind.

Meditation to Open the Heart Chakra

Sit in a comfortable, cross-legged position. The mantra is SAT KAARTAAR (*a* as in "bus"; *aa* as in "far"). As you say SAT, the hands are pressed together at the center of the chest in **prayer mudra (a).** As you say KAAR- the arms are extending out in front of you with hands and fingers pointed straight up **(b).** As you say -TAAR the arms are moving out to the sides parallel to the floor, fingers still pointed up **(c).** Make the transition from step to step in a flowing movement. *Duration of meditation: 3, 11, 31, or 62 min.*

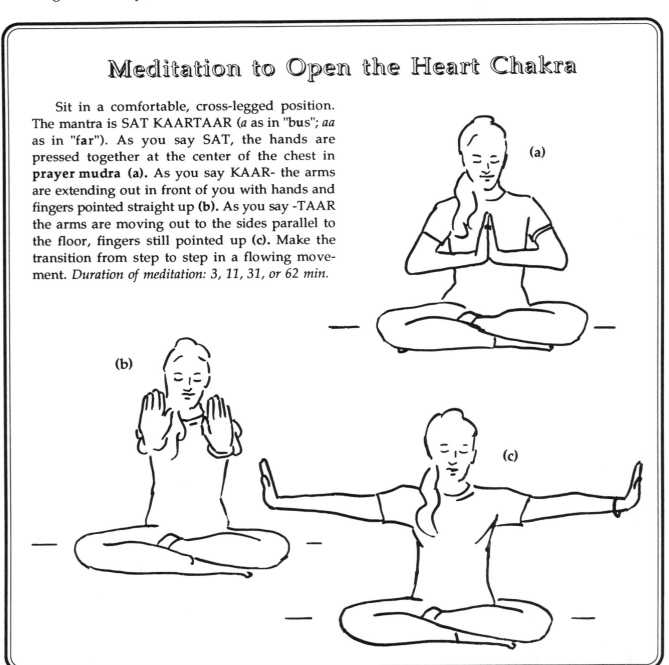

The Pineal Gland

Ancient scientists from both western and eastern cultures seem to have been aware of the extraordinary nature of the pineal gland. The Greek anatomist Herophilus identified the gland as a precondition for higher thought, referring to it as a "sphincter" that regulates the flow of thought. Yogis refer to it as the location of the seventh, or **crown chakra,** and called it the **tenth gate.** To them, it was the door of perception. In human beings, this tiny piece of body tissue that sits at the juncture of the spinal cord and the brain looks like a small wilted mushroom. Yogis (and more recently, Western scientists) have related the pineal gland to sexual function, nerve and muscular strength, magnetic field strength, and extrasensory perception. Obviously, it is an area of great importance to students of kundalini yoga.

In the late 1940s, an important discovery was made about the pineal gland. Scientists, working on a number of independent research projects, isolated a secretion called **serotonin.** Serotonin was found to regulate muscle action in the walls of the intestines and to help in the clotting and flow of blood and in the action of smooth muscle tissue. More importantly, it was found to act as an agent that opened the mind to perception of alternate realities. These discoveries led to increased research on hallucinogenic drugs and altered states of consciousness. It was found that yogis were actually able to increase the production of serotonin in the brain, part of the process that led to the experience of the **meditative mind,** what most Westerners know as the religious experience.

This was not news to yogis, who for years had been eating foods such as figs, bananas, and banyan sap, all of which are rich in serotonin and stimulate the pineal gland. The image of the Buddha sitting under the banyan tree is directly symbolic of the power and importance of the pineal gland.[2]

----

[2]Onions, ginger, and garlic, when linked to a regular kundalini yoga practice, also help increase the activity of the pineal gland.

Yoga and meditation[3] transform the spinal fluid to a more highly concentrated form, called **"ojas,"** causing the pineal gland to secrete. Scientists are now beginning to recognize the pineal gland as a sense organ that reacts to, and is highly affected by, light. This discovery has made scientists reconsider the concept of extrasensory perception. They are now beginning to concede that we do, indeed, have the sense mechanisms to perceive higher realms of consciousness and what has heretofore been called psychic energy.

Kundalini

Over Shiva Linga shines the sleeping Kundalini, fine as the fiber of the lotus stalk. She is Maya in this world, gently covering the hollow on the head of Shiva Linga. Like the spiral of a conch shell, her shining snakelike form coils three and a half times around Shiva Linga, and her luster is that of a strong flash of young lightning. . . .

By meditating on the Kundalini, which shines within the root chakra with the lustre of 10 million suns, a man becomes Lord of Speech, king among men, and an adept in all kinds of learning. He becomes ever free from all diseases, and his inmost spirit becomes full of great gladness. Pure of disposition, by his deep and musical words he serves the foremost of the gods.

—Purananda of Bengal

Kundalini energy is experienced when the energy of the glandular system combines with that of the nervous system to create such a sensitivity that the brain as a whole receives signals and integrates them. The autonomic and voluntary nervous systems come under conscious control, allowing a person to become completely aware of himself and his environment. The kundalini energy is the creative potential of everyone; in its experience lies the realization of that potential.

----

[3]The "Addiction" meditation in Chapter 4 stimulates and balances the pineal gland.

9

Some say that mankind once lived in total God-consciousness. Between man and God there was no difference, except that man was manifest on this earth and God was unmanifest. Then man turned from God-consciousness to **maya,** the illusion of the senses, so God separated man's consciousness into two halves. One half man uses to live his earthly life, but the higher consciousness remains sleeping until man evolves far enough to be able to use it again. The story of Adam and Eve might be said to represent this fall from grace, the garden of Eden being a state of total awareness, the apple representing maya, and the serpent representing kundalini, divine knowledge.

In fact, the kundalini energy has often been called **"serpent power,"** a name whose sinister implications hardly do justice to the benign reality of this energy field. The yogis of India regard it as the embodiment of **"Adi Shakti,"** the primal creative power. It is the energy that developed us, gave us the shape we have, and brought us on earth. It is pure energy, without residue. The word itself is sometimes translated "coil of the beloved's hair." In its dormant state, it lies coiled at the base of the spine.

In a functional sense, all that needs to be done to activate the kundalini is to uncoil this energy and connect it with the pineal gland at the top of our heads, which after a child reaches 8 years of age normally ceases to secrete fully. When that master gland, the "seat of the soul," taps the energy of the kundalini, it will begin to secrete as it did when we were young. This is the state called "kundalini risen"; some call it enlightenment.

Awakening the Kundalini

The process by which this unfolding occurs is complex. The kundalini will not awaken and rise until two energies are integrated and balanced. These two forces are **apana** and **prana.** Apana is an eliminating force; it affects functions operating on both gross and subtle levels in the body to expel negative energy and waste. In reference to the process of raising the kun-

dalini, it might be considered the "vital air" below the navel.

Prana is the "vital air" above the navel. The life force penetrating every atom of our form, and indeed, of the universe, is stored in our bodies at the **eighth thoracic vertebra,** the part of the spine located near the bottom edge of the shoulder blades. This pranic center, by means of the **"pranic nerve,"** enervates a U-shaped muscle responsible for autonomic nervous system function—heartbeat, movement of the diaphragm, responses beyond our conscious control. The ancient yogis could create pranic energy reservoirs at the **"pranic cavity"** and live on that reserve.

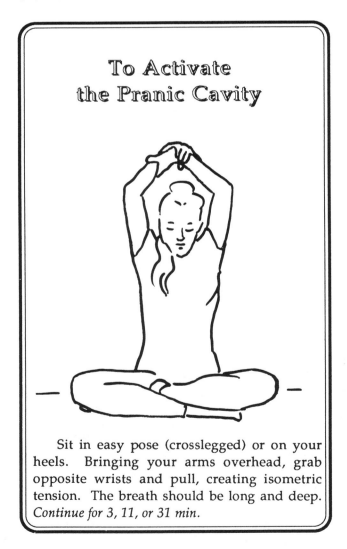

To Activate the Pranic Cavity

Sit in easy pose (crosslegged) or on your heels. Bringing your arms overhead, grab opposite wrists and pull, creating isometric tension. The breath should be long and deep. *Continue for 3, 11, or 31 min.*

To stimulate the kundalini, one must inhale and hold the breath, directing prana down to the navel point. Then one exhales and "holds the breath out" (i.e., refrains from inhaling), drawing apana up from the base of the spine to the navel point. When prana and apana meet and unite, a tremendous "white heat" or **"tapa"** is created at the navel point.[4] The combined energies are often described as the filament of **sushumna ("silver cord")**, a nerve current or **nadi** thought by some to correspond to the governor vessel meridian of Chinese medical theory, and by others to correspond to the central nervous system of Western medical theory. When the energies combine, this sushumna lights up like the filament in a light bulb suddenly plugged into its source of electric power. Responding to breath control and mental direction, the integrated energies depart the navel point and descend to the base of the spine, where they stimulate the dormant kundalini. Further breath control and the application of the will cause the force to rise, along with the kundalini power, charging the higher centers of consciousness, the chakras. In this way a person's energy can be transmuted into higher forms.

Nadis

There are 72,000 main nerve currents, or nadis, which emanate from the navel point and end in the hands and feet. Through these nadis, which are said by some to correspond to the cardiovascular and lymphatic vessels, and by others to correspond to acupressure meridians, prana is carried to all parts of the body. The ida, pingala, and sushumna are the three most important nadis. The ida and pingala come from the left and right nostrils, respectively, and travel down the spine, crossing at the various chakras along the spine. The sushumna originates from the base of the spine, where the three main nadis meet, and travels up the center of the spine to the top of the head.

----

[4]For exercises to create tapa see the **Yoga Manual** (Appendix C).

In order for the kundalini energy to flow, certain blocks and impurities in the nadis must be removed; the channels must be cleansed. This can be done using breath and mantra in conjunction with various postures and **"body locks."**

Raising Kundalini Energy

When the prana–apana descend to the base of the spine, they place the kundalini under pressure to expand and rise. The kundalini is like oil placed under pressure; the various body locks (see also the section "Body Locks" in Chapter 2) are used to raise the kundalini and the prana–apana up from the lower chakras and send them up the sushumna. Pressure in the root, or first, chakra sends the force up to the navel point. This pressure is called **"root lock."** Application of **"diaphragm lock"** sends it up towards the fifth, or throat chakra. From there **"neck lock"** takes it to the brain. In order to stimulate the pineal gland (the "seat of the soul") the tenth gate (crown chakra), located at the top of the head, must be "unsealed." When the kundalini heat rises, the pineal is said to radiate toward the pituitary gland along a channel called the **"golden cord,"** which responds with colored pulses. When both glands are activated, the third ventricle of the brain— the **"third-eye point,"** the gate to the crown (seventh) chakra—opens.

While the process for awakening the kundalini is simple, the force involved is most powerful. Therefore, two cautions: first, always hold your spine completely straight as you apply the locks. Pull your neck slightly in (not down or up), like the British royal guard. That way there will be as little bend in the neck as possible. If your spine is not quite straight, the energy circuit will not be complete. Second, as a beginner, practice the three locks under the guidance of a kundalini yoga teacher (see Appendix B). If there are none in your area, be sure to chant the words **"ONG NAMO, GUROO DEV NAMO"** (see the section on "Tuning In" in Chapter 2) three times before beginning, so as to tune in to your own higher consciousness to guide you through the process.

Sat Kriya to Raise the Kundalini

Sat Kriya is probably the most powerful **kriya** (yoga exercise) in the science of kundalini yoga. With regular practice, it increases the lung capacity, perfects the functioning of all the body organs, stimulates circulation, generates and raises great energy, and brings the experience of kundalini energy rising up the spine.

Before practicing this kriya, be sure to "tune in" (Chapter 1). Next, sitting on the heels, with a straight spine, stretch the arms straight up overhead, hugging the ears. If you are a beginner, interlace the fingers, with only the index fingers pressed together and pointing straight up. Advanced students can place palms together, all fingers of both hands touching and pointing straight up. The eyes are closed and focused at a point midway between and slightly above the eyebrows, about 1/4 inch inside the skull (the **third-eye point**).

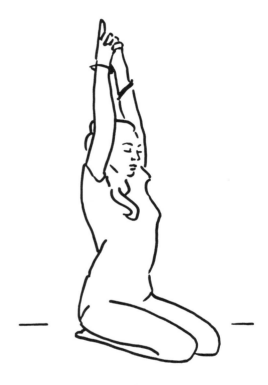

Chant the sound SAT (*a* as in "**bus**") from the navel point as you pull root lock (pull up and in on the rectum, sex organs, and navel point). Then release the lock as you chant NAAM (*aa* as in "**far**"). The breath will come automatically. The shoulders will naturally rise up an inch or two as the lock is pulled. The spine does not flex.

Continue for 3-31 min. Then inhale and exhale long and deep several times. On the last exhalation, hold the air out and apply root lock, diaphragm lock, and neck lock (Chapter 2). Focus on drawing energy up the spine to the third-eye

point. Inhale. Repeat the breathing exercise and the locks once or twice if you wish. Then relax out of the posture.

Lie down on your back, arms resting along your sides, and relax. *Be sure to allow at least as much time for this relaxation as you took to do the kriya.*

2. BASICS OF YOGA

Doing kundalini yoga is a little like taking medicine—if you don't take the proper dose, or if you take the wrong kind of "medicine" for your particular difficulty, you won't achieve the required results. It's important to follow directions precisely as to length of time to do the technique, exactly how to do the technique—taking into consideration breath, posture, sequence of postures, body locks, and so on—and to do so in a quiet, undistracting environment. It's a good idea to become familiar with the explanations in this chapter before you begin your practice, so that you will be generally familiar with the terms used in the remaining chapters. Then refer back to this chapter for specific techniques as they are mentioned later, until you are quite sure your technique is right. It is also a very good idea to attend yoga classes at a kundalini yoga teaching center (see Appendix B) so that you can get feedback from a teacher already familiar with the techniques.

Kriyas

A kriya is one or more exercises and/or meditation(s) that produce a specific state of mind and body. Doing a kriya initiates a sequence of physical and mental events that affect the mind, body, and spirit simultaneously. The effects of each kriya are well marked, often manifold,[1] and often very different from those of every other kriya.

Every form of exercise is not a kriya. To shift gears in a car you do not randomly push the clutch, pump the gas, and move the gear shift lever. To change gears, you must sequentially go through each step and you must coordinate the engine speed, the clutch, and the proper sequence of changing gear ratios. Similarly, to shift the state of consciousness a number of systems, both physical and mental, must be stimulated and coordinated to create a stable change. Kriyas code these particular combinations in a subtle way and control how the various energy systems interlock. Therefore, when you come upon a set of exercises in this book, make sure you practice the set as specified. Do each part in the stated order and as well as you can. Relax where relaxation is specified. Be meticulous—this yoga is a science, and you are a great scientist, performing the most significant experiment in life—that of transforming yourself into the healthy, happy, divine being that you, in essence, already are.

----

[1]For instance, **"frog pose"** (see "Postures," this chapter) is good for the heart, hearing, and eyesight; flushes the arteries and lymph system; strengthens and transforms sexual energy for use in the higher chakras; and helps prevent breast cancer and tennis elbow.

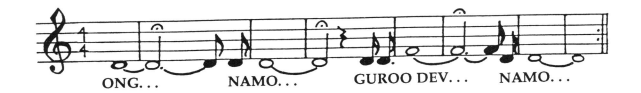

ONG... NAMO... GUROO DEV... NAMO...

Tuning In

Every kundalini yoga practice should begin with chanting the **Adi Mantra**: ONG NAMO, GUROO DEV NAMO. By chanting it in proper form and consciousness, the student humbles himself before his higher self, the source of all guidance, and opens the protective link between himself and the divine teacher within.

How to Recite the Adi Mantra

Sit in a comfortable, cross-legged posture with a straight spine. Press the palms of the hands together at the center of the chest with the fingers pointed straight up **(prayer pose)**. Draw the hands tightly into the chest so that the joints of the thumbs are pressed against the sternum (the place where the two halves of the rib cage meet).

Inhale deeply. Focus your concentration at the third-eye point, midway between the eyebrows, about 1/4 inch up and 1/4 inch in. As you exhale, chant the words ONG NAMO, using the entire breath to produce the sound. Then take a quick sip of air through the mouth and chant the rest of the mantra, GUROO DEV NAMO, extending the sound as long as possible. The sound DEV is chanted a minor third higher than the other sounds of the mantra. (For relative pitch and rhythm, see the musical notation below.) As you chant, vibrate the cranium with the sound so that a mild pressure is felt at the third-eye point. Chant this mantra 3 times before beginning your yoga practice.

How to Pronounce the Adi Mantra

The *o* sound in ONG is long, as in "hope" and of relatively short duration. The *ng* sound is relatively long and nasal and produces a definite vibration on the roof of the mouth and in the cranium. The *a* in NAMO is like the *u* in "bus." The *o*, as in "hope," is held for a long time. The *u* in the word GUROO is pronounced as in the word "good." The *oo* is pronounced as in the word "mood." The first syllable, therefore, is short and the second one long. The *e* in DEV is like the *a* in "gate."

What This Mantra Means

ONG is the infinite creative energy experienced in manifestation and activity. It is a variation of the cosmic syllable OM, which is used to denote God in His absolute or unmanifested state. When God creates and functions as Creator, He is called ONG.

NAMO has the same root as the word NAMASTE, which means "reverent greetings." In India, NAMASTE is a common form of respectful greeting spoken while one's palms are pressed together at the chest or forehead. It implies bowing down. Taken together, the words ONG NAMO mean "I call on the infinite creative consciousness," opening myself to the universal consciousness that guides all action.

GUROO is the teacher or embodiment of the wisdom that one is seeking. DEV means "divine" or "of God," in a nonearthly, transparent sense. NAMO, in closing the mantra, reaffirms

14

the humble reverence of the devotee. Taken to-gether, GUROO DEV NAMO means "I call on the divine wisdom," I bow before my higher self to guide me in using the knowledge and energy given by my unlimited essence.

Mental Focus

For each technique described in this manual, you will find the appropriate postures, finger positions, body locks, breathing patterns, and movements specified. One ingredient that is not always specified is mental focus. Generally speaking, unless directed to do otherwise, you should fix your concentration on the third-eye point, a point midway between the eyebrows, 1/4 inch up and 1/4 inch inside the head. With your eyes closed, you can mentally locate this point by turning your eyes gently upwards and inwards. Concentration at the third-eye point does not mean blocking out all other awareness. Remain aware of your breath, your body posture, your movements, and any mantra you may be using, but make your center of awareness your third-eye point.

Breath Techniques

Kundalini yoga employs a wide range of breathing techniques. They are more extensive and sophisticated than in any other form of yoga. The breath, its rhythm, and its depth correlate to different states of health, consciousness, and emotion. Kundalini yoga uses the breath to change the body's energy state. There are several basic breaths that should be mastered in order to freely practice kundalini yoga.

Long, Deep Breathing

Long, deep breathing is the simplest of all yogic breaths. It is the breath you had as a child, the kind of breath that animals do, and that to which people in primitive societies are still attuned. Unfortunately, due to stress, most adults in our culture have lost the knack for it.

Benefits. If you can re-educate your body to do long, deep breathing, your health will improve in many ways. You will feel relaxed and calm. Your magnetic field will be revitalized, making you less liable to fall victim to accidents, sickness, and negativity. Toxic buildup caused by not clearing the mucous linings of the alveoli (small cavities) of the lungs will be reduced. The blood will be cleansed, and the increased oxygen flow to your brain and body will speed up both emotional and physical healing. Long, deep breathing also rechannels previous mental conditioning on pain (as, for example, in childbirth) so as to reduce or eliminate the sensation of pain.

How to do long, deep breathing. Relax your chest and shoulders. Inhale, relaxing the abdomen, or even pushing it out (a). The muscles of the abdomen will draw down the diaphragm, a circular barrier of muscular tissue separating the lung cavity from the abdominal cavity. The downward movement of the diaphragm will create a vacuum in the lung cavity, so air will automatically flow into the lungs. Think of a big pitcher slowly filling with water—like your lungs becoming filled with air, starting at the bottom, and slowly filling to the top. Then as you exhale, rather than contracting the chest, allow the abdomen to shrink back in, or try pulling it in at first (b). This pushes up on the diaphragm, creating a pressure in the lung cavity, causing air to be expelled.

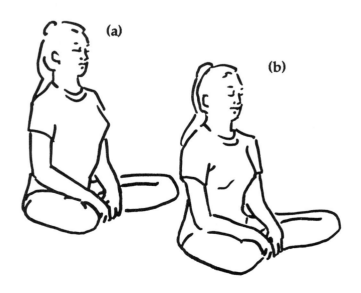

Go at this technique very wholeheartedly. Normally people use only 600-700 cubic centimeters of their 6,000-cubic-centimeter lung capacity when they breathe. Even if you think you are breathing very deeply, just relax, open up, and free up the breath more than you thought possible. To check yourself at first, you may wish to place one hand on the abdomen. That way you can feel the abdomen expanding as you inhale and contracting as you exhale.

Breath of Fire

In this breath, which is used frequently in kundalini yoga, the focus of energy is at the navel point. The breath is fairly rapid (2 to 3 breaths per second), continuous, and powerful, with no pause between the inhalation and the exhalation. The mouth is closed unless otherwise specified. As you exhale, the air is pushed out as the navel point and abdomen are pulled in towards the spine. In this motion the chest area stays moderately relaxed. You should feel the pull of the muscles in the area of the navel. As you inhale, the abdomen relaxes, the diaphragm extends down, and the breath seems to come in as part of relaxation rather than through effort.

When you first begin to practice this breath, you may find that your inhalation is more emphasized than your exhalation, or vice versa. As you become familiar with the technique, strive for a very balanced breath, with no emphasis on either the inhalation or the exhalation, giving equal power to both.

Breath of fire should be practiced with a closed mouth, as the restricted flow of air through the nostrils prevents hyperventilation. This breathing technique should be mastered slowly and methodically, as it causes an immediate detoxification reaction in the body. Old toxins and deposits from drugs, smoking, and bad nutrition are released from the lungs, mucous lining, blood vessels, and cells. These toxins leave the body through the blood and lymphatic systems. As a result of this cleansing process, you may feel temporarily lightheaded or queasy as you practice the breathing tech-

nique. If this happens, relax for a while and allow the kidneys to filter out the toxins. To aid the cleansing process, drink plenty of water, increase the amount of exercise you do each day, and simplify your diet to light vegetables, fruits, and nuts for a few weeks.

Benefits. Breath of fire is said to cleanse the entire blood supply of the body in 3 min. It raises the voltage of the nervous system and strengthens shaky nerves. Besides releasing toxins, it expands the lung capacity and strengthens the magnetic field, as does long, deep breathing. It can also help overcome addictions and cleanse you of the bad effects of smoking, taking drugs, and consuming sugar, alcohol, and caffeine.

Other Breaths

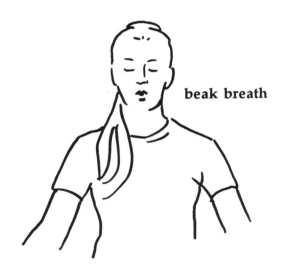

beak breath

Beak breath. Beak breath is used with only a few kriyas, such as Vatskar Kriya. The mouth is pursed in a tight *o*, like a beak. The breath is inhaled, either in one long stroke or in short sips (the description of the exercise should indicate whether long or short), through the "beak" and exhaled through the nose.

16

Broken breaths. This technique divides the inhalation and exhalation into parts or "strokes" according to a specific ratio. Each ratio has a different effect. Some typical ratios for the series "inhale, hold air in, exhale, hold air out" are 4:0:4:0, 3:0:1:0, 4:0:1:0, and 1:8:1:8.

Let us consider the 4:0:1:0 ratio (more commonly known as 4:1). This breath is one of those used to heal oneself and to break out of depression. The inhalation is broken into 4 equal strokes. Each part is a quick sniff-like inhalation through the nose that causes the sides of the nose to collapse in slightly. When the last stroke of the inhalation is completed, the lungs should be **completely** expanded. Care must be taken to make the strokes of equal duration, while still ending up with the lungs completely expanded. Then one exhales in a single, long breath through the nose, expelling the last tiny bit of air from the lungs as the exhalation is completed. The exhalation must be very complete, so that the inhalation begins with empty lungs. Focus on the breath throughout; make the technique as perfect as possible.

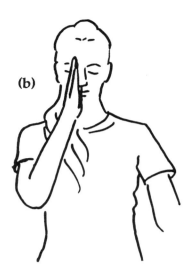

Left nostril breathing. With the thumb of the right hand, block the right nostril (b). The fingers of the right hand are together and pointing straight up. Breathe as indicated in the exercise, through the left nostril only.

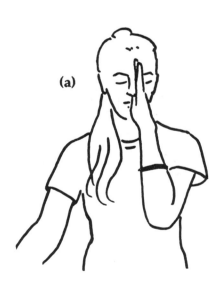

Right nostril breathing. With the thumb of the left hand, block the left nostril (a). The fingers of the left hand are together, pointing straight up. Breathe in whatever way the exercise indicates, through the right nostril only.

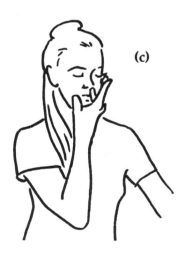

Alternate nostril breath. Block alternate nostrils, one with the little finger and the other with the thumb of the same hand, as you inhale through one nostril and exhale through the other (c). If the exercise description does not specify, inhale through whichever nostril you prefer, and exhale through the other.

Unspecified Breath

When a breathing technique is unspecified in a rhythmic exercise, become aware of the position of your lungs during parts of the exercise. In parts of the exercise where the lungs tend to expand, inhale. In parts of the exercise where the lungs are constricted, exhale. For example, if you are doing an exercise where you stand up, hands stretched back overhead, then bend over and touch palms to the floor, you will naturally want to inhale as hands go up and back, and exhale as your chest is constricted and palms are on the floor (d). In **spine flex,** where you sit in a comfortable, straight-spine position and the spine is flexed forward and back, you will want to inhale as the spine flexes forward, a position that allows the lungs to expand naturally. When the spine flexes back and the chest is somewhat constricted, you will want to exhale (e).

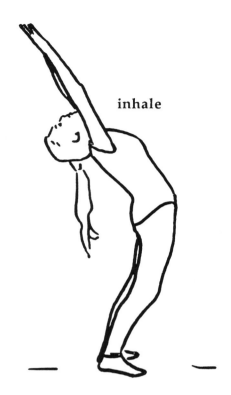

inhale

(d) touching toes

exhale

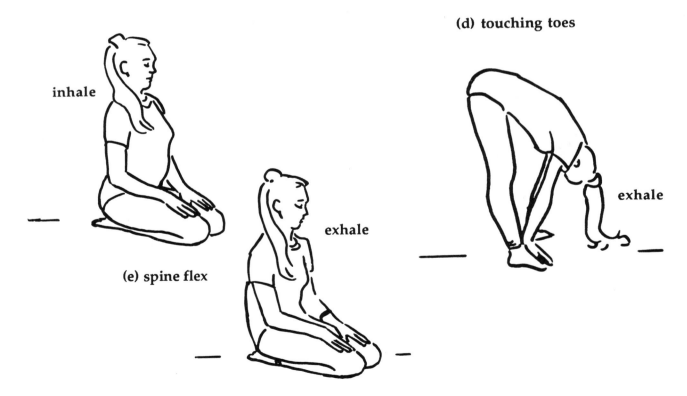

inhale

(e) spine flex

exhale

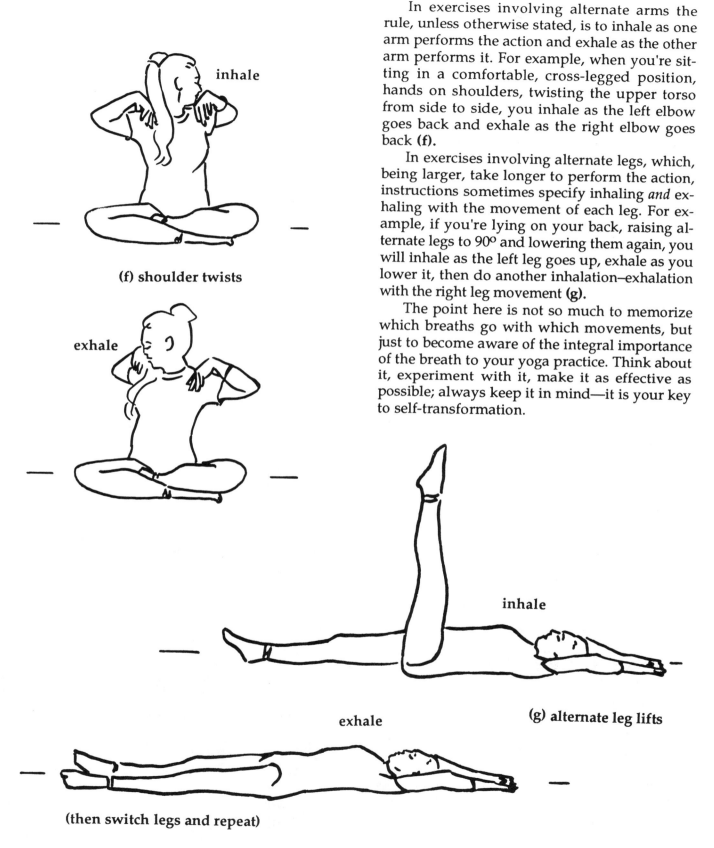

inhale

(f) shoulder twists

exhale

In exercises involving alternate arms the rule, unless otherwise stated, is to inhale as one arm performs the action and exhale as the other arm performs it. For example, when you're sitting in a comfortable, cross-legged position, hands on shoulders, twisting the upper torso from side to side, you inhale as the left elbow goes back and exhale as the right elbow goes back **(f)**.

In exercises involving alternate legs, which, being larger, take longer to perform the action, instructions sometimes specify inhaling *and* exhaling with the movement of each leg. For example, if you're lying on your back, raising alternate legs to 90° and lowering them again, you will inhale as the left leg goes up, exhale as you lower it, then do another inhalation–exhalation with the right leg movement **(g)**.

The point here is not so much to memorize which breaths go with which movements, but just to become aware of the integral importance of the breath to your yoga practice. Think about it, experiment with it, make it as effective as possible; always keep it in mind—it is your key to self-transformation.

inhale

exhale

(g) alternate leg lifts

(then switch legs and repeat)

Mantras

EK ONG KAAR-A, SAAT-AA NAAM-A, SEE-REE WHAA-A-HE GUROO. This is the laya yoga form of the **Adi Shakti Mantra**. The rhythm of the chant gives it a sense of "spinning" that rotates the energy of the chakras and the aura. The effect is one of total absorption in Infinity. "There is one Creator who has created this creation. Truth is His Name. Great beyond words is the ecstasy of His wisdom."

ONG NAMO, GUROO DEV NAMO. ONG is pronounced far back on the palate, and resonated in the nose. This is the **Adi Mantra**: "I bow to the Infinite creative consciousness, to the Divine Teacher within." To be chanted three times before doing yoga.

ONG SOHUNG. ONG is pronounced far back on the palate, and resonated in the nose, as is HUNG. HUNG is pronounced as in English. "O God the Creator, I am Thou."

RAA MAA DAA SAA. RAA means "sun," MAA "moon," DAA "earth," and SAA "infinity."

RAA MAA DAA SAA, SAA SE-EE SOHUNG (HUNG is pronounced as in English) The **Siri**

Gaitri Mantra: "I am that balance between sun and moon, earth and ether." Literally: "Sun, moon, earth, infinity, that totality of Infinity is Thou, I am Thou."

RAA RAA RAA RAA, MAA MAA MAA MAA, SAA TAA NAA MAA. "Sun (RAA), moon (MAA), infinity (SAA), birth (TAA), death (NAA), rebirth (MAA)." The sound of this mantra travels the mental orbit of our lives.

SAA TAA NAA MAA . This is the **bij**, or **seed mantra** SAT NAAM broken down into its nuclear form of five primal sounds: *s, t, n, m,* and *a*. The syllables mean "infinity, birth, death, rebirth." The totality includes both finite and infinite.

SAT KAARTAAR. "True Doer."

SAT NAAM. "Truth is the Name, is the identity."

WAAHE GUROO. The **Mantra of Ecstasy**: WAAHE is an untranslatable expression of one experiencing the Creator's supreme power. It is ecstasy. GUROO means wisdom, the sense of higher wisdom.

Notes on Pronunciation: Vowels in the Gurmukhi transliterations in this list and throughout this manual are pronounced as follows: *a* as in "bus," *aa* as in "far," *ai* as in "elder" or "cat," *au* as in "claw" or "sound," *e* as in "gate," *ee* as in "see," *i* as in "sit," *o* as in "hope," *oo* as in "mood," and *u* as in "good." The cassette tape "Mantras for Meditation" by Krishna Kaur Khalsa, available from Golden Temple Enterprises, Box 13, Shady Lane, Espanola, NM 87532 (phone 505-753-0563), demonstrates the pronunciation of most of these mantras.

Linking Breath with Mantra

One aspect of kundalini yoga that is frequently unspecified is the use of mantra. A mantra is a series of sounds, generally having an inspirational meaning such as a name of God, the rhythmical repetition of which can be used to elevate or modify consciousness. We have already seen how the mantra ONG NAMO, GUROO DEV NAMO is used to tune the mind in to its own higher consciousness before practicing kundalini yoga. Other mantras, each having its own qualities, rhythm, and effects, are specified with various exercises and meditations.

It is beneficial throughout the practice of kundalini yoga to utilize the power of mantra by linking a mantra to the breath even when no mantra is formally specified. The mantra most commonly used is **SAT NAAM** (rhymes with "but Mom"). SAT NAAM means "truth is my identity." This mantra can be linked with the breath by mentally repeating SAT as you inhale and mentally repeating NAAM as you exhale.

Another good mantra is **WAAHE GUROO.** WAAHE is an expression of ecstasy; it should be mentally repeated on inhaling. GUROO means "divine inner teacher"; it should be mentally repeated on exhaling.

In linking one of these mantras to the breath, you filter your thoughts, making sure that each thought chain has a positive resolution. You will also find that the use of a mantra makes it easier to keep up in the performance of any exercise that is particularly strenuous and that it adds depth to the performance of even the simplest exercise.

Most beneficial of all is to carry the practice of mantra into your daily life. As you are doing chores, walking, or driving, you can chant or sing your mantra. As you are resting or working listen to chants on tape.[2] The more you do the chant, mentally or aloud, the calmer your mind will become, and the more relaxed you will feel. Your breathing will deepen and your awareness of yourself and your surroundings increase as mind and body tune in to the flow of all that is.

Postures

Each exercise of a kundalini kriya specifies what position to take. Sometimes the instructions for a posture simply state that you should sit in a comfortable, cross-legged posture, with a straight spine. If you can't sit that way comfortably, it's all right to sit on a small, firm pillow to keep the spine straight. If your muscles are very stiff and the posture must be held for a

---

[2]Four excellent chants available on cassette tape from Golden Temple Enterprises, Box 13, Shady Lane, Espanola, NM 87532 (phone 505-753-0563) are "Aap Sahaee Hoaa" by Singh Kaur and Amar Singh Khalsa, "Naad: The Blessing" by Sangeet Kaur, "Rakhe Rakhan Hara" by Singh Kaur Khalsa, and "Narayan" by Sat Peter Singh Khalsa.

long time, you may need to sit in **rock pose** (see below) or on a chair instead. Whatever your sitting position, it is important to feel balanced and stable. If you lean to one side or have great pain in your knees or ankles, you cannot meditate properly. If you meditate in an off-balance posture, you run the risk of misdirecting the energy and blood circulation that are stimulated by the technique. Your sitting posture should always feel well-balanced and comfortable to you. It should reflect harmony.

Easy Pose (Sukasana)

There are 3 variations of **easy pose** to choose from:

1. Sit with the legs out straight. Pull one foot in next to the groin. Place the other foot over the ankle of the first foot so that it rests near the thigh. Straighten the spine **(a).**

2. This is like the first variation, but the top foot is placed on the calf of the other leg, rather than right at the groin. In this pose, make sure to press the lower spine forward, as it will have a tendency to slip backward.

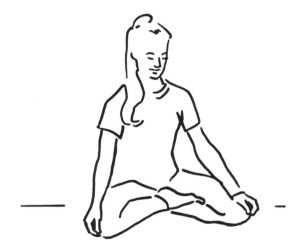

(a) Upper foot may rest on opposite ankle or opposite calf.

21

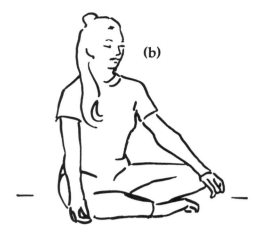

(b)

3. If the first two postures are too rigorous, try this one. Sit up with both legs straight. Put one foot under the opposite knee and then draw the extended foot under the other knee. Pull the spine up straight and press the lower spine slightly forward **(b).**

All these variations of easy pose are easier on the knees and require less flexibility than lotus pose. The drawback is that one must be more conscious of keeping the lower spine slightly forward so the upper spine can stay straight.

Lotus Pose

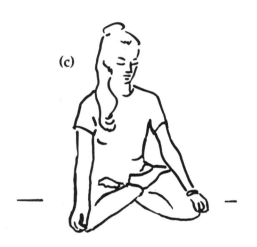

(c)

Sit with the legs extended forward. Spread the legs. Bend the left leg so the left heel comes to the groin. Lift the left foot onto the upper right thigh. Bend the right leg so that the right foot rests on top of the left thigh as close to the abdomen as possible **(c).** Straighten the spine. Lift the chest and press the lower spine slightly forward. This position will feel "locked in place." Once you are in it you can meditate very deeply and the position will maintain itself.

Although very few exercises or meditations require this difficult posture, it is recognized as one of the best postures for deep meditation.

Rock Pose (Vajrasana)

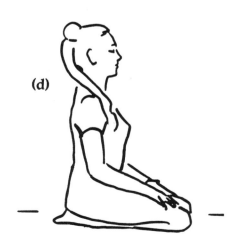

(d)

This posture is well known for its beneficial effects on the digestive system. It gained its nickname from the idea that one who masters the posture can sit in it and "digest rocks." It also makes you solid and balanced as a rock.

To get in the position, start by kneeling on both knees, with the tops of the feet on the ground. Sit back on the heels. The heels will press two nerves that run into the lower center of each buttock. Keep the spine pulled straight **(d).**

22

Half Lotus

There are two poses frequently referred to as the half-lotus position. The easier one is a variation of easy pose. Sit in easy pose. Pull the top foot all the way across onto the upper thigh **(e)** instead of leaving it on or under the opposite leg.

The other half lotus is a little more difficult. Sit in rock pose and then stretch the right leg out straight. Bend the right leg so the foot rests on the upper left thigh. You are sitting and balancing on the left heel and the right knee **(f)**. When specifically indicated in the instructions, the pose may be done with the legs switched.

Perfect Pose (Siddhasana)

This posture is excellent for stimulating the nervous system and utilizing the body's sexual energy. It requires practice to perfect, but once it is mastered, simply sitting in this posture puts you into meditation.

Extend both legs straight. Bend the right leg and put the toes of the right foot in back of the left knee. Next, bring the left heel under the right leg and under the sex organ. The left heel should touch the spot on the pelvis between the sex organ and the rectum. The toes of the right foot are contained in the bend of the left knee. Only the big toe is exposed. Pull the spine straight **(g)**.

When you first begin to practice this posture, do it for a few minutes only, building up gradually to as long as you like.

Celibate Pose

Sit with your heels just to either side of your buttocks. Hands can be in any of a number of positions **(h)**.

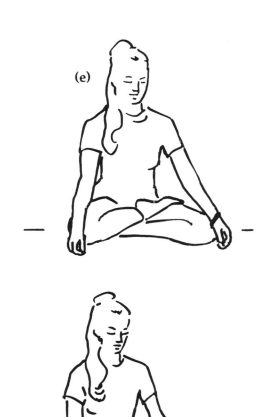

(f) sitting on left heel

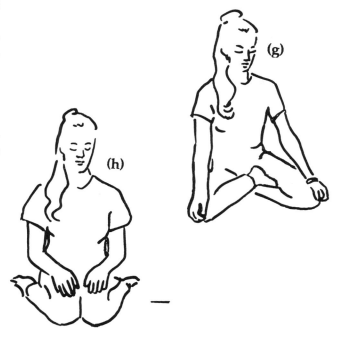

Sitting in a Chair

If none of these poses is comfortable for meditation, you may sit in a chair **(i)**. Pick a chair that gives you firm support. A large, over-stuffed lounge chair may be uncomfortable for a long meditation. The back of the chair can give you support if it is straight.

Most people have a tendency to totally relax or slump in a chair. Such an impulse can be countered by reminding yourself that you are sitting down to become relaxed and totally attentive.

A common error lies in letting the legs hang loosely. It is essential that the feet be placed squarely on the ground, so that the lower spine and hips do not get out of balance.

Corpse Pose

Lie down on your back, arms along your sides, hands palms up **(j)**.

Crow Pose

There are several variations of this pose. One involves squatting on the haunches, feet flat on the floor, with hands clasped round the knees, fingers interlocked **(k)**.

A more dynamic variation involves inhaling as you rise up into a standing position with the arms straight out in front of you, palms down **(l)**, then exhaling as you sink down to a position squatting on the haunches, feet flat on the floor, with arms still straight out, palms down **(m)**.

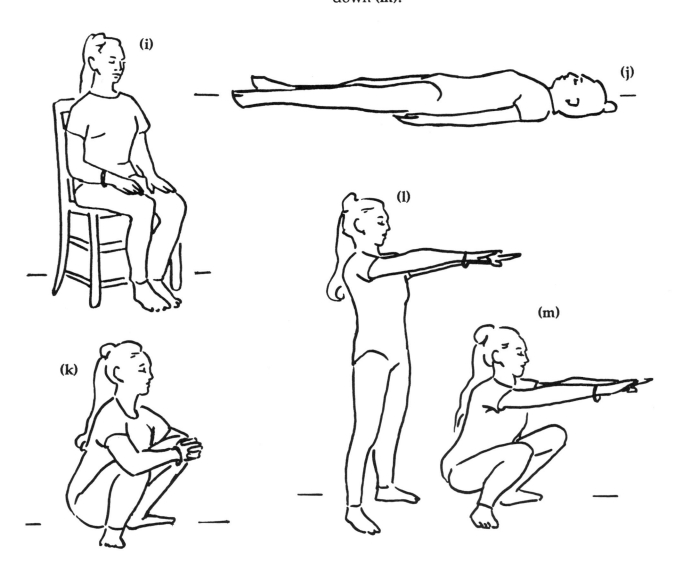

24

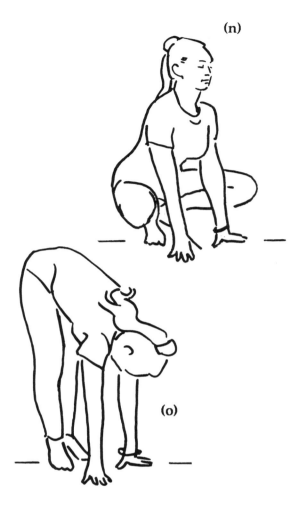

(n)

(o)

Frog Pose

Frog pose is another 2-part exercise. As you exhale, you sink into a squatting position, with buttocks on heels, knees spread wide, heels together and off the ground, and toes spread wide for balance. The arms are between the knees, fingertips on the floor. At the end of this sinking movement the head is up, facing straight forward **(n).** As you inhale, raise the buttocks high, taking care to keep the fingertips on the ground and the heels together and off the ground throughout. At the end of the rising movement, the head faces the knees **(o).** With your next exhalation, return to the original position, coming down forcefully enough that the buttocks strikes the heels sharply.

Maha Mudra

Sit on the left heel, stretch the right leg forward, and grab the big toe of the right foot with the right hand. Pulling back on the toe, grab the heel of the right foot with the left hand. Keep the back straight, the chin tucked into the chest, and the eyes fixed on the big toe **(p).**

This mudra usually involves pulling root lock, the exact sequence of motions being specified with the individual exercise involved.

Stretch Pose

Lie down on your back, hands along your sides, palms down, fingers together. Raise the legs till the heels are 6 inches off the ground, toes pointed forward. Also raise the head and hands 6 inches off the ground **(q).** Take care to keep the small of the back on the ground throughout the exercise, as in so doing the abdominal rather than the lower back muscles are strengthened.

This exercise sets the navel point and strengthens the abdominal muscles. It is usually done with breath of fire, or sometimes with long, deep breathing.

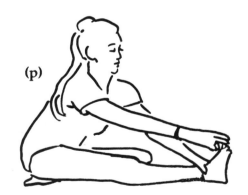

(p)

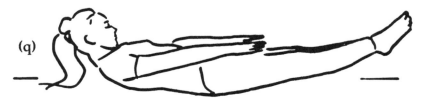

(q)

Mudras (Finger Positions)

Early in life we use our hands in our first exploration of the world as we learn to manipulate it. The hand expresses our moods in each minute gesture. If you look at the palm, you will see that the lines form intriguing patterns. If you understand the coding, the hands are an energy map of our consciousness and health. Early yogis mapped out the hand areas and their associated reflexes. Each area of the hand reflexes to a certain area of the body or brain. Each area also represents different emotions or behaviors. By curling, crossing, stretching, and touching fingers to other fingers and areas of the hand we can effectively talk to the body and mind. The hands become a keyboard for input to our mind/body computer. Each **mudra**, or finger position, listed below is a technique for giving clear messages to the mind/body energy system.

Gyan Mudra

This mudra is said to bring knowledge to the ego. There are two forms: for **receptive gyan mudra**, put the tip of the thumb together with the tip of the index finger. The other fingers are extended and joined **(a)**. For **active gyan mudra**, bend the index finger under the thumb so the fingernail is on the terminal joint of the thumb **(b)**. Unless otherwise specified, use the first variation.

Venus Lock

This mudra channels sexual energy and balances glands. Interlock the fingers, left little finger on the outside of the hand. Men should have the right thumb on the outside of the hand, and women should have the left thumb on the outside. The outside thumb should press down firmly on the pad below the inside thumb. The inside thumb should press into the webbing between the forefinger and thumb of the opposite hand **(c)**.

Prayer Mudra

This mudra is always used when tuning in before doing kundalini yoga. Place both hands flat together, fingers together **(d)**. This neutralizes the positive (right, or male) and negative (left, or female) sides of the body.

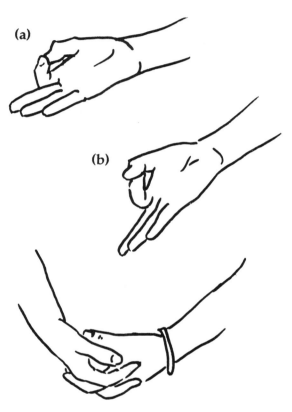

(c) Venus lock (for women).
For men, the thumbs are reversed.

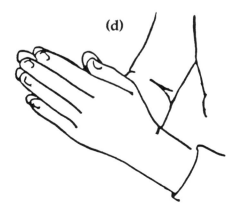

Bear Grip

This mudra is used to stimulate the heart and to intensify concentration. Place the left palm facing out from the chest with the thumb down. Place the palm of the right hand facing the chest. Lock the fingers of each hand into the fingers of the other hand (e).

Buddha Mudra

Another fairly common mudra for meditation is formed by placing the right hand palm up in the left palm. [For women the palms are reversed—(f).] The thumbs are pressed together and forward. Sometimes the mudra is placed in the lap, sometimes just beneath the breasts.

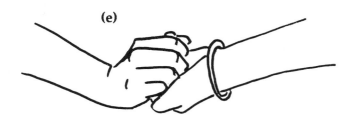

(e)

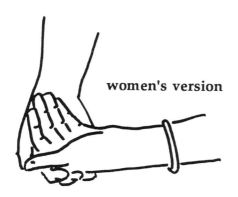

women's version

(f) Buddha mudra

Body Locks

Certain combinations of muscle contractions, called body locks or **bhandas,** are frequently applied in kundalini yoga. These locks change blood circulation, nerve pressure, and the flow of cerebrospinal fluid. They also direct the flow of prana, or life force, into the nadis, or energy channels, through which the kundalini energy flows. They concentrate the body's energy to raise the consciousness and bring about self-healing. There are 3 important locks: **neck lock, diaphragm lock,** and **root lock.** When all 3 are applied simultaneously, the combination is called **maha bhand,** the **great lock** of kundalini yoga.

Neck Lock

The most basic lock used in kundalini yoga is neck lock, or **jalandhara bhand.** This lock is practiced by pulling the head back in toward the neck, without tilting the head up or down. The effect is rather like that of the British royal guard standing at attention. This action straightens the bones of the neck, allowing pranic energy to travel freely into the glandular centers of the brain. It also keeps the blood pressure steady when the kundalini rises, so that you don't get dizzy or feel uncomfortable pressure in the head. Pressure is placed on the thyroid and parathyroid glands, regulating their secretion and activating the consciousness-expanding functions of the pituitary. If the lock is not applied, breathing exercises can cause uncomfortable pressure in the eyes, ears, and heart.

As a general rule, apply neck lock in all meditations unless instructions indicate otherwise.

Diaphragm Lock

This lock, otherwise known as **uddiyana bhand,** is often applied rhythmically during chanting. Lift the diaphragm up high into the thorax (the chest area) and pull the upper abdominal muscles back toward the spine. This creates a cavity that gives a gentle massage to the heart muscles **(a).** Diaphragm lock allows prana to travel through the sushumna, or central pranic channel, up into the neck region. It is also directly involved in stimulating the hypothalamic–pituitary–adrenal axis in the brain. It stimulates one's sense of compassion and can give new youthfulness to the entire body.

Note: Keep the spine straight. Apply the lock only on exhaling, as untoward pressure is created in the eyes and heart if the lock is applied forcefully on inhaling.

Root Lock

The most complex of the locks, root lock or **mul bhand,** is frequently called for in kundalini yoga exercises. Root lock coordinates, stimulates, and balances the energies of the rectum, sex organs, and navel point. Roughly speaking, it is performed in 3 motions. The first is to contract the sphincter muscle of the anus, drawing it in and up, as if trying to prevent a bowel movement. Next, contract the sex organs, drawing them up as if attempting to stem the flow of urine through the urethral tract. Last, contract the navel or abdominal muscles toward the spine. The 3 actions are performed in a smooth, flowing, rapid manner, almost simultaneously **(b).** It helps to visualize energy coursing from the rectum up through the navel point as you pull the lock.

The actual physical trigger points of root lock are slightly different in men and women. A man should try to contract the root chakra located in the perineum between the anus and the sex organs. For a woman, the contraction should begin at the cervix, where the vagina and uterus meet. Try to locate the exact point for your gender, and begin contracting there. Then

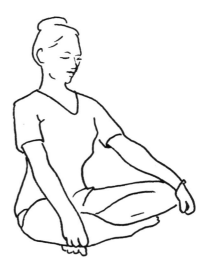

(a) Diaphragm lock on a complete exhalation. The lock creates a vacuum effect in the abdominal cavity and neck area.

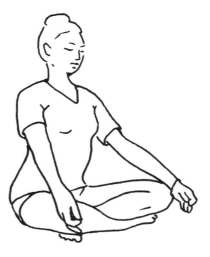

(b) Root lock being done on a complete inhalation. Note the expansion of the rib cage created by contracting the abdominal muscles toward the spine.

28

immediately contract the navel point. If in doubt, use the 3-part contraction method until you become more aware of the exact point of contraction.

The root lock performs two functions: It simultaneously draws apana, or "eliminating" energy (which usually flows downward in the body), up to the navel center and draws prana, the "vital air," down to the navel center. There the two energies merge, generating psychic heat. This heat, or tapa, descends to the root chakra, releasing the kundalini energy. Hindu sacred scriptures describe it thus:

"Contract the perineum firmly. Draw the apana upwards. When the apana and the fire meet at the navel chakra, the prana is heated. This increases the digestive fire. Due to the kindling of this fire—apana and prana—the sleeping kundalini is awakened."

Note: This lock is applied on the held exhalation unless otherwise specified.

Maha Bhand, the Great Lock

Maha bhand (*a*'s as in **far**) is the simultaneous application of all 3 locks—root lock, diaphragm lock, and neck lock. Visualize energy coursing up the chakras as you pull the locks almost simultaneously, from lowest to highest. This practice rejuvenates the nerves, glands and chakras. It regulates blood pressure, reduces menstrual cramps, and puts extra blood circulation into the lower glands (testes, ovaries, prostate, Cowper's glands, Skene's gland, etc.).

Pacing Yourself

Many kundalini kriyas involve rhythmical movement between two or more postures. In such cases the pace at which you should move is generally not stated. As a rule, you should begin slowly, keeping a steady rhythm. Increase gradually, being careful not to strain. Generally speaking, the more you practice an exercise, the faster you will find yourself able to go, but in any case, be sure that the spine has become warm and flexible before attempting rapid movement.

Concluding an Exercise

Unless otherwise stated, an exercise should be concluded by inhaling and holding the breath briefly, then exhaling and, while maintaining the posture, applying root lock on the held exhalation. This helps to consolidate the effects of any exercise and to circulate the energy to the higher centers of the body. How long the breath should be retained depends upon your level of accomplishment as a student. More experienced students with highly developed lung capacities can hold their breath for longer periods of time than can most beginning students. In no case, however, should you hold the breath to the point of passing out. If you start to feel dizzy, immediately inhale and relax.

Relaxation

An important part of any exercise is the relaxation following it. Unless instructions specify otherwise, allow 1-3 min of relaxation in a comfortable and convenient posture, generally in easy pose, corpse pose (relaxed on the back), or lying flat on the stomach, after each exercise. The less experienced you are in the practice of kundalini yoga and the more strenuous the exercise, the longer the relaxation period that will be required. During **sadhana,** or early morning spiritual practice, when the body is normally relaxed to begin with, it may be necessary to reduce relaxation time to a bare minimum so as to remain awake. At other times, if a period of "deep relaxation" is specified after an exercise, you may rest for 3-10 min. Always end your yoga practice with such a relaxation.

Concluding a Set of Exercises

After a long relaxation, particularly one that follows a set of exercises, you will find that doing the concluding exercises below will help ground you and bring you back to reality:

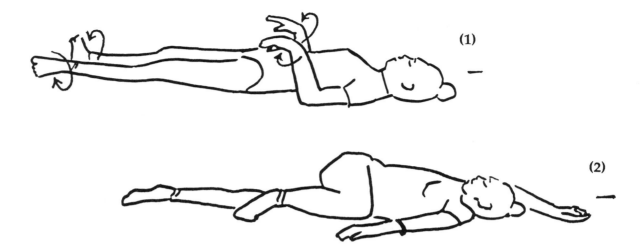

1. On your back, begin rotating your feet and hands in small circles. Continue in one direction for half a minute, then in the other direction for another half minute.

2. **Cat stretch:** Keeping both shoulders and the left leg flat on the ground, bring the right arm back behind the head and the right knee over the left leg till it touches the floor on the far side of the body. Switch legs and arms and repeat the exercise.

3. Still on your back, bring the knees up and to the sides, and rub the soles of the feet and the palms of the hands together briskly, creating a sensation of heat. Continue for a minute.

4. Clasping knees to chest with both hands, begin rolling on the spine. Roll all the way back till the feet touch the ground behind the head, and all the way forward till you're sitting up. Do this 3 or 4 times.

5. Sit up in easy pose, palms together in prayer mudra at the fourth chakra, or **heart center.** Eyes are closed. Sing to yourself the "Longtime Sunshine" song (see below) 3 times.

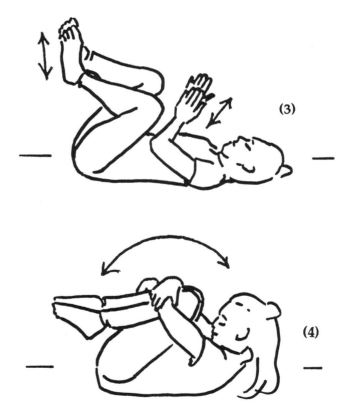

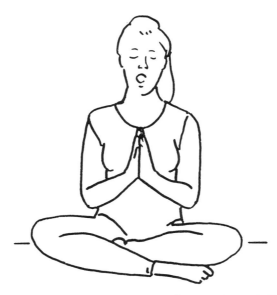

LONGTIME SUNSHINE SONG

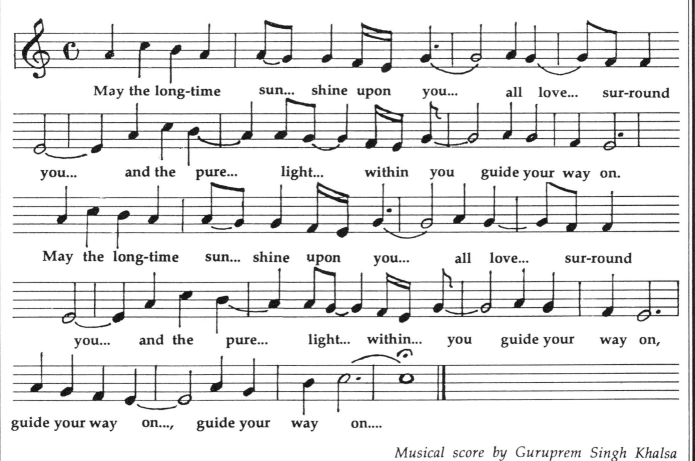

May the long-time sun... shine upon you... all love... sur-round you... and the pure... light... within you guide your way on.

May the long-time sun... shine upon you... all love... sur-round you... and the pure... light... within... you guide your way on, guide your way on..., guide your way on....

Musical score by Guruprem Singh Khalsa

31

3. STAYING HEALTHY

As modern health care plans are beginning to acknowledge, by far the most effective way to treat disease is to prevent its occurring at all. While all yoga has the effect of bolstering health, some exercises and meditations (see Chapter 4) are very specific in their disease-preventive and/or therapeutic effects. Other kriyas, such as those at the end of this chapter, have the general effect of increasing the body's ability to resist disease. If you tend to be ill a lot, or if you feel an undefined illness coming on, these are excellent kriyas to do. But first let's explore some key areas of the body, attention to which is vital to good health.

KEY AREAS IN THE BODY

Shoulders

Stay tuned in to your body's telltale signs—stiffness in the shoulders, especially at the acupressure points located near the spine, just off and down from the tops of the shoulder blades **(a)**. According to **The Yellow Emperor's Classic of Internal Medicine** (written over 4,000 years ago), wind and cold enter the pores of the skin at these points. In ancient India as well, stiffness in the shoulder blades was considered to contribute to illness. It was a practice in India to swing a thick branch or club back and forth to break down the tension. You can do the same with a baseball bat, or you can open up the energy flow in the area with **yoga mudra**:

Sit on your heels, grasping your hands in Venus lock behind the back. bring the forehead to the floor and stretch the clasped hands up to the ceiling **(b)**. Hold this position with long, deep breathing *for at least 3 min.*

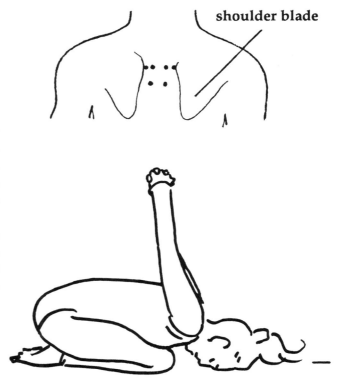

shoulder blade

The Feet

The feet are a strong center of prana (life force) and of electromagnetic field (auric) activity. Kirlian photography indicates that the feet balance out the human aura. Also, nerve endings in the feet reach to every part of the body and affect the health of the body as a whole. That's why foot care is very important to health. A natural way to take care of your feet is to walk barefoot on soft dirt or sand. This will stimulate and massage them. But walking on asphalt, concrete, and other hard, flat, artificial surfaces is bad for your feet. It breaks down their natural structure and causes calluses and crystals to form. So wear shoes when walking on unnaturally hard surfaces.

Choose shoes that give firm support and do not constrict the shape of the feet. Flat shoes molded to the contour of the foot (such as Birkenstocks or Shakti Shoes) are best. High heels deform the feet and throw the spine and pelvis out.

Remove dead and callused skin by soaking in warm water and then using a pumice stone. Massage oil into them every day. Wash them morning and night with cold water and rub with a coarse, dry towel to help stimulate nerve activity and to keep the feet sensitive.

Because of their sensitivity and special relationship to the rest of the body, the feet can tell you a lot about the health of the body as a whole. A pain in the foot that is not related to direct injury there is a sign that the body is about to become ill. The area of the foot that hurts indicates the area of the body affected. (See foot chart below.) Foot massage on such points is an excellent form of preventive care.

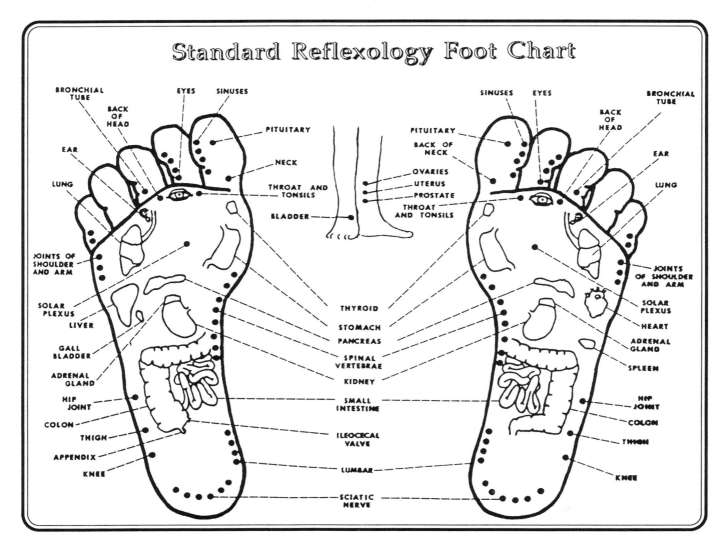

Standard Reflexology Foot Chart

34

How to Massage a Foot

You will need a bottle of massage oil (almond oil or coconut oil are best) and a coarse bath towel. Have the person to be massaged lie down and cover them with a blanket. Rub massage oil into one foot; keep the bottle within reach in case you need it later.

First ask the person what problems they are having with their foot; if there are areas (such as cuts or injuries) you should avoid or treat gently. Then, following the foot chart, begin at the top of the foot and progress downward using short upward strokes about an inch long. Use the thumb, or, for extra pressure, the knuckle. How hard you press depends on the sensitivity of the person you're working on and the part of the foot involved. Most people can't take much pressure on the arch of the foot; the heel, however, generally requires knuckle work.

When you reach a trouble area—perhaps a hard spot (calcium deposit, sometimes called a "crystal") under the skin, or you may sense a slight change of temperature or a tiny jolt of energy, or the person may just tell you the area hurts when you press—make a mental note of it and, after you cover the entire foot, return and work on that area. Have consideration for your "patient's" state of mind. Foot massage is therapeutic, but it should not be so painful that your friend will never want another one. It must, however, be firm enough that calcium deposits will, over the course of several treatments, begin to be broken down and energy flow to the related organ stimulated.

After the first foot is finished, rub it with the towel and then wrap it with one end of the towel, leaving enough towel to rub and wrap the other foot later. Do the other foot. Make sure your friend is warm and comfortable. (They will probably be asleep.) See that they don't get up for at least the length of time that they were massaged.

After you finish, shake your hands vigorously in the air to discharge your friend's magnetic field from your own. Wash your hands and wrists in cold water to prevent "transference" of their symptoms to yourself.

Onion Massage

In cases of a high fever that must be brought down rapidly, or if the body is very toxic, massage the feet with half an onion. It does sound strange, but it helps.

Breathing and the Lungs

It is in the lungs that the breath of God kisses man's body. They are our interface with the divine energy of the universe. In a physical sense, the lungs supply oxygen to the blood and life force, or prana to the body. Air pollution, smoking, and improper breathing hinder this health-giving process.

Air pollution is a health factor that can only be dealt with by such large measures as political action or choice of living location. But smoking is a factor directly within our reach. If you would like to quit smoking, practice the "Addiction" meditation (Chapter 4).

Just as important as either of the above is the question of proper breathing. The average person breathes about 15 times a minute under normal conditions. A practiced yogi breathes about 8 times a minute. To develop a truly meditative mind, you must reduce the breath to less than 4 times a minute.

Without sustained deep breathing, the breath does not reach the deeper parts of the lungs. As a result, the blood is improperly purified. This leads to thickening of the arteries and clogged capillaries. The magnetic field is diminished, the nerves become weak, and the body wears out and loses its resistance to disease.

Indian lore holds that each person is allotted at birth a specific number of breaths. (Most people today breathe a total of about 600,000,000 times.) It was felt that if a person breathed more slowly he would use up his quota more slowly, hence live longer. Whether or not this is so, it is true that those who breathe more deeply and more slowly are less prone to hypertension, heart disease, nervous tension, digestive disorders, and other diseases.

For general health and longevity, it is important to practice long, deep breathing (Chapter 2) consciously all the time. Breath of fire, also described in that chapter, will remove impurities from the blood and lungs. Tradition has it that from the beginning to the end of one session of breath of fire—whether it is for 1 min or for 10—is just 1 "breath," so there is no need to worry about using up your quota quickly. If you do 10 min each of left nostril breathing, right nostril breathing, breath of fire, and long, deep breathing (Chapter 2) consecutively, the entire blood supply will be cleansed several times.

The Liver

As will be mentioned in discussing "Diet" (Appendix A), a healthy liver is essential to overall well-being. The liver manufactures, cleanses, and proportions the ingredients of the blood. Its malfunction causes death. Meats, oily foods, eggs, poorly cooked or rancid foods, chemicals, and preservatives all tax the liver. Alcohol and overeating are the most active agents in its destruction.

If you don't have a serious liver disorder, such as hepatitis, see Chapter 4 for a good liver-strengthening exercise. Cleansing juice diets will also help heal an abused liver. Particularly recommended are beet juice diluted with water (taken straight, it can make you ill), or a mixture of 3 parts carrot juice to 1 part daikon radish juice. During the first few days of the fast, when toxins from the liver are jettisoned into the bloodstream, you will feel a little high and giddy. After the toxins are eliminated, you'll begin to feel a wonderful, healthful feeling you may not have felt since you were a child. But please be careful: Consult your yoga teacher or health practitioner before fasting, don't fast for more than 3-4 days at a time, and don't drink too much beet juice. A few ounces a day are enough.

The Navel Point

Between the navel and the last bone of the spinal column is the navel center, shaped like a bird's egg. Within it is the starting point of the 72,000 nerves, of which 72 are vital. Of these again 10 are most important. In order to have proper control over these 10 nerves, one has to take special pains.

—*Upanishads*

Masters of the martial arts have known for centuries of the unique nature of the navel point as the center for power and balance in the body. By mastering it they were able to perform remarkable physical feats. In Chinese acupressure, this "shinketsu" point is thought to be the place where divine energy flows in and out of the body. To Indian yogis, the navel point is known as the Mother Energy Point, a point of power and balance at which prana enters the body from other dimensions. It is also a springboard from which they can ascend into the higher realms of meditation.

It is the navel center which ensures that the 72,000 nerves and arteries spread over the entire body perform their assigned tasks satisfactorily. We take many precautions to keep the body free of disease—we feed it, exercise it, treat it with medicine when necessary. But if the navel center is off balance, all these efforts are in vain.

Let's do an experiment. Lie down on your back and, placing the thumb and fingers of one hand together **(a)**, press them firmly but gently down into the navel. Somewhere near the navel you will feel a strong pulse. If this pulse is ex-

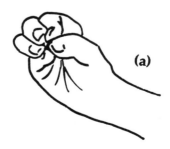

(a)

actly at the navel, the navel point is said to be centered. This state is best for your health. If the navel point pulse is off center, many hard-to-diagnose maladies can result. Displacement of the navel upward, for example, is associated with constipation, acid blood, heart disease, and general irritation. Displacement downward causes colic pain and bad dreams. Lateral displacement leads to acute pain that is difficult to alleviate with drugs. Among women, displacement can lead to such problems as leukorrhea and menstrual irregularity; they may have children that are weak and short-lived, or they may be barren.

Fortunately, simple exercises are available to center the navel. One such is **stretch pose:** Lie down on your back. Place the heels together, point the toes forward, and lift the heels 6 inches off the floor. Raise the head to the same height, eyes focused on the toes. Arms are off the floor, not touching the hips, with palms towards the body and fingertips towards the toes

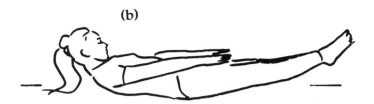

(b)

(b). Begin breath of fire (Chapter 2) for 1 min. Then inhale, hold the breath in for 15 seconds, and relax down. You can build the time up to 3 min with practice.

Daily practice of stretch pose will bring the navel point back into balance. As this happens, you should also feel renewed poise, power, and inner strength.[1]

----

[1]For more information on and exercises for the navel point, see the **Meditation Manual,** pp. 5-19 (Appendix C).

YOGA SETS
FOR GENERAL HEALTH MAINTENANCE

If you feel yourself on the verge of getting ill, practice one of the following yoga sets.

KRIYA TO PREVENT SICKNESS
(about 30 min)

1. Sit in easy pose, right hand in gyan mudra resting on your right knee. Block the left nostril with the thumb of the left hand. Have the fingers of the left hand together, straight, and pointed up. Begin long, deep, powerful breaths through the right nostril. *Continue for 3-5 min,* then inhale, exhale, and relax.

2. Sit on your heels in rock pose. Stretch your arms up, elbows hugging ears, palms together overhead. Begin **Sat Kriya.** The mantra is SAT NAAM (rhymes with "but Mom"). Chant the sound SAT from the navel point as you pull root lock and pull the navel point in sharply. Chant the sound NAAM as you relax the lock and the navel. *Continue for 3 min.* Then inhale and pull energy up from the anus all the way through the top of the skull (maha bhand). *Now relax for 1 min.*

Repeat all of Exercise 2, including the relaxation, 2 more times.

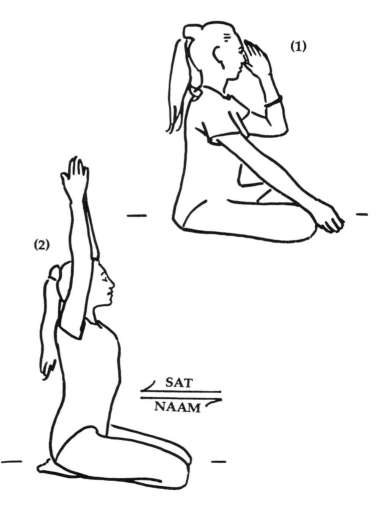

(1)

(2)

SAT
NAAM

38

3. Sit in easy pose, grasping your shins with both hands. Inhale deeply as you flex the spine forward **(a)**, mentally saying the word SAT. Exhale completely as you allow the spine to collapse back **(b)**, mentally saying NAAM. Keep the head level throughout.

Continue rhythmically with deep breaths *108 times*, applying root lock with each exhalation. When you finish, inhale and hold briefly with the spine perfectly straight. Relax.

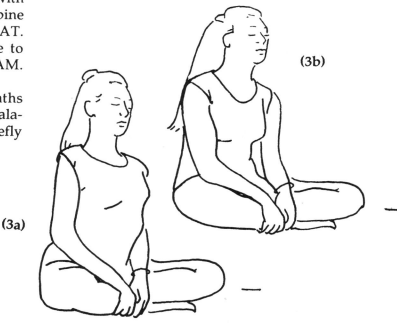

(3b)

(3a)

4. Come into **frog pose:** Squat down so the buttocks are on your heels. The heels are off the floor and touching each other. Put the fingertips on the floor between the knees. Keep the head up **(a).** Inhale and raise the buttocks high, keeping the fingertips on the floor and the heels together and off the floor. At the height of the inhalation, the head is facing the knees **(b).** Then exhale back down to the original position, letting the buttocks strike the heels. The exhalation should be strong. Continue with deep breaths *a total of 26 times*.

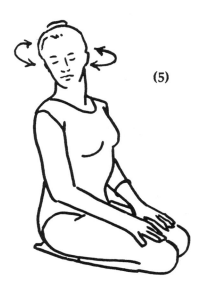

(5)

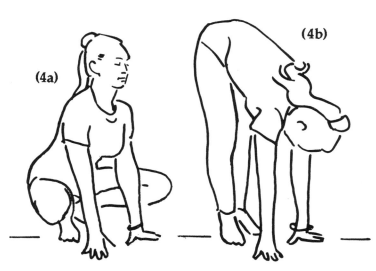

(4b)

(4a)

5. Sit on your heels, hands on the thighs. With the spine very straight, turn your head to the left as you mentally say SAT. Exhale as you turn your head to the right, mentally saying NAAM. *Continue for 1-3 min.* Then inhale with the head straight forward, and relax.

6. Sit in easy pose and put the hands on the shoulders, thumbs in back. The upper arms are parallel to the floor **(a)**. Inhale and bend to your left **(b)**, then exhale and bend to the right. Keep the upper arms in a straight line throughout. Continue this swaying motion with deep breaths *for 3 min.* Then inhale straight and relax.

7. Sit in easy pose with a straight spine. Direct your attention through the third-eye point. Pull in on the navel point and up on root lock and hold them so. Watch the flow of the breath. As you inhale, listen to silent SAT. As you exhale, listen to NAAM silently. *Continue for at least 6 min.*

Comments

This is an excellent set of exercises to help the beginning student of yoga prevent sickness. The set is named **Surya Kriya** after what is known in yogic lore as "sun energy." It is an energy of purification. It holds the weight down, aids digestion, and makes the mind clear, analytical, and action-oriented. Exercise 1 creates a clear, focused mind. Exercise 2 releases the kundalini energy stored at the navel point for your use. Exercise 3 brings this kundalini energy up the spine and aids digestion. Exercise 4 transforms the sexual energy for use in the higher chakras. Exercise 5 stimulates circulation to the head and the thyroid and parathyroid glands. Exercise 6 distributes energy to the body as a whole and balances the magnetic field. Exercise 7 takes you into a deep, self-healing meditation.

The overall effect of the kriya is to stimulate prana and the kundalini in your body. Regular practice will make your body strong and your mind energetic, expressive, and enthusiastic.

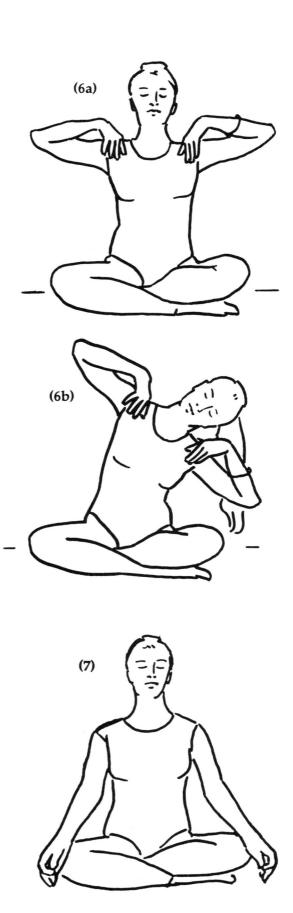

(6a)

(6b)

(7)

FOR A STRONG, ENERGETIC BODY
(up to about 15 min)

1. Sit up, legs out straight in front of you, hands on the floor beside the knees. Inhale deeply. Exhale completely, then inhale again. Hold the breath in, press the toes forward, and lift the legs up to 60º. The breath should be held in for from 20 seconds to 1 min, depending on your capacity, and never more than 3 min under any circumstance. Exhale and relax. *Do this exercise a total of 10 times.*

2. Sit as before, legs out straight. Look at the tip of your toes. Keep the spine as erect as possible—90º—and lift the legs up to 60º, arms out straight in front, hands next to the knees. Inhale completely. In a monotone, chant over and over again as you exhale: SAT NAAM, SAT NAAM, SAT NAAM, SAT NAAM. . . . Feel the sound come from your navel point.

Continue for 1-3 min. Relax. *Then repeat all of Exercise 2.*

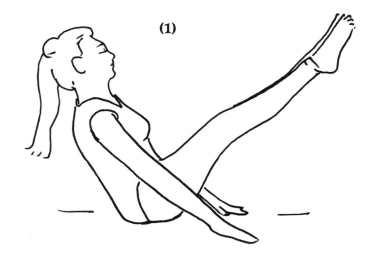

(2)

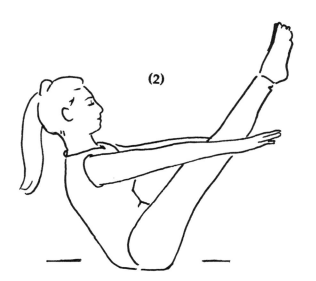

(1)

Comments

These moderately difficult exercises are famed for their recuperative quality. The first, **Maha Shakti Kriya,** is described in Indian scriptures thus: "Hold your own breath, and the breath will become the nectar of life. Death will run away from you." If you feel old, diseased and unhappy, go into a quiet room and do this kriya. Do it with an attitude of love and devotion.

The second exercise generates tremendous energy. It stimulates the life force to such an extent that it can even aid heart patients.

These exercises will make your body shake with exertion, but it is really better to have the body shake now than in old age. After you finish the set you will feel full of energy, so that you will not need pills to keep it going.

VARUYAS KRIYA
FOR HEALTH AND LONG LIFE
(3-15 min)

Stand up straight. Put the right foot slightly forward. Stretch the left leg far backward. Put the top of the toes of the left foot on the floor behind you. Place the hands in prayer mudra at your chest (or extend the arms, palms together, straight out in front of you). Tilt the spine slightly forward from the vertical. Fix the eyes either on the horizon or at the third-eye point.

Take a deep breath, then begin rhythmically chanting SAT NAAM over and over. Emphasize the sound SAT as you pull the navel point in and apply a light root lock. *Continue for 1 1/2 min.* Then inhale and relax.

Switch legs and repeat the exercise for an equal period of time.

Comments

This difficult kriya will test your will power and nerve strength. It will make you sweat if you do it properly. You may also notice a burning sensation in the cheeks. The time of practice can slowly be increased to 7 1/2 min on each side.

Regular practice and perfection of this kriya has extensive positive effects on the body. It increases general immunity to disease, strengthens the nervous system, rebalances the body's magnetic field, transmutes sexual energy to the higher chakras, and enhances the function of the pituitary gland. It has the same "shake now, but not in old age" effect as the kriya "For a Strong, Energetic Body."

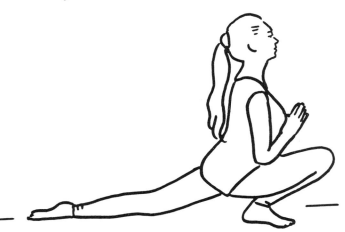

Varuyas Kriya - arms may also be stretched straight out in front, palms together

42

REJUVENATION MEDITATION
(11-31 min)

Sit in easy pose with a straight spine. With elbows relaxed, bring hands, palms up, to heart level, little fingers of the two hands touching along their length. Other fingers and thumbs are spread apart. Look at the tip of your nose, and beyond that deeply into the earth.

Deeply inhale through a semi-puckered mouth and hold the breath in for 4-5 seconds. Then completely exhale all the air from the lungs in 4 **equal** breaths though the nose, mentally saying SAA TAA NAA MAA on the 4 strokes. Hold the breath out for 2-3 seconds, then continue the cycle.

Begin by practicing *for 11 min*. Very slowly build your practice to 31 min; under no circumstances should the meditation be done for more than 31 min.

Comments

This is a very powerful meditation. Working mainly on the glandular system, it produces strong health and excellent regenerative capabilities. It is best done **just before bed,** as you will feel spaced out afterwards. If you do it during the day, **be sure to give yourself adequate time to recover from it,** so as not to jar the nervous system. Otherwise, you may undo all the good you have done for yourself through its practice!

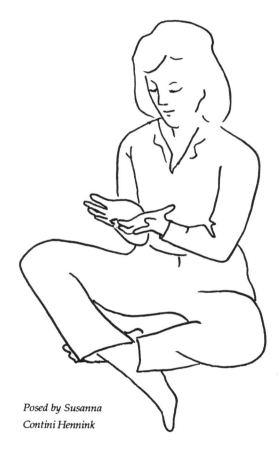

Posed by Susanna Contini Hennink

43

FOR FURTHER REFERENCE

For a meditation to bolster the immune system, which protects your body's overall health, see the entry "Blood Cells, to Balance Red and White," in Chapter 4. A set of exercises to avoid persistent colds and illness, for physical strength, and for increased disease resistance can be found in **Keeping Up with Kundalini Yoga,** pp. 23-25. An energizing and healing meditation for women only can be found in **Slim and Trim,** p. 25. The **Survival Kit** contains a meditation said to bring health and healing ability, to eliminate fatigue and depression, and to give a constant flow of energy (p. 12). The **Yoga Manual** contains a set of rather difficult exercises for body cleansing and disease prevention (pp. 30-34). These are especially good for women, but are recommended for men as well. The **Sadhana Guidelines** contains a set to prevent disease by strengthening the aura (p. 59) and a set for disease resistance and to strengthen the heart (p. 65). See Appendix C for more information.

4. HEALING THE SELF

Abdomen, Weak
(1-3 min)

Lie on your back. Inhale and raise both legs up to 90° **(a).** Exhale and lower the legs **(b).** Continue rhythmically with powerful breathing *for 1-3 min.*

Comments
Lack of abdominal strength is often a source of **lower back pain,** as the muscles of the lower back are overworked attempting to compensate.

For an abdominal strengthening set, see **Sadhana Guidelines,** pp. 57-58.

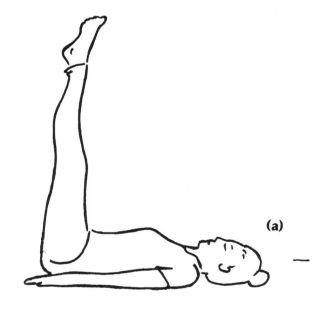

(a)

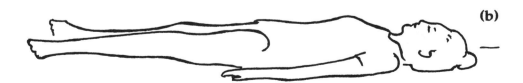

(b)

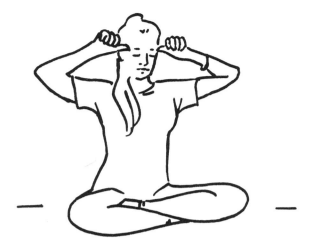

Addiction
(5-7 min)

Sit in easy pose with a straight spine, making sure that the lowest 6 vertebrae are pushed forward. Make fists of the hands. Extend the thumbs straight and place them on the temples in the niche where they fit. Lock the back molars and keep the lips closed. Vibrate the jaw muscles by alternating the pressure on the molars. A muscle will move in rhythm under the thumbs. Feel it massage the thumbs as you apply a firm pressure with the thumbs.

Keep the eyes closed. Look to the third-eye point. Mentally vibrate the mantra SAA TAA NAA MAA (*aa*'s as in "far") at the third-eye point. (See staff below.)

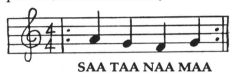

SAA TAA NAA MAA

Continue for 5-7 min. The time may be expanded to 20-31 min with practice.

Comments
This "Medical Meditation for Habituation" is effective in overcoming such physical addictions as **smoking, overeating, alcohol,** and **drugs.** It also works on **subconscious addictions** which lead us to insecure and neurotic behavior patterns, and on **phobic conditions.**

Adjustments, Ankles and Knees
(1-2 min)

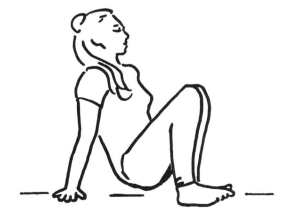

Sit down. Draw your knees to your chest, feet on the floor. Place the hands on the floor at the sides of the body and balance the entire body weight on the hands and heels. *Hold the position for 1-2 min.*

Adjustments, Elbows
(3 min)

Sit in lotus pose if you are able. If not, sit in easy pose with tightly crossed legs. Make fists and put the knuckles on the floor at the sides of the body. Use the arms to raise the body 3-6 inches, then drop it. *Continue for 3 min.*

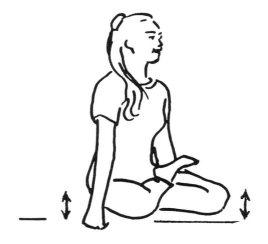

Adjustments, Feet
(1-2 min)

To adjust the toes and balls of the feet, sit with a straight spine, knees firmly held into the chest by the arms. Rock forward in an effort to get onto the feet. Although this will not be possible, in the effort to do so the appropriate muscular tension will be created.
Continue for 1-2 min.

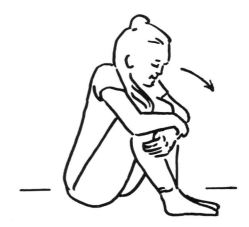

Adjustments, Hand
(5 min)

To adjust the bones of the hand, sit in easy pose. Bring the hands together in front of the chest with only the fingertips touching. Keeping the fingers straight, press the palms out as the hands rotate out and away from the chest, and in as the hands come toward the chest. The hands will rotate in small circles.
Continue for 5 min.

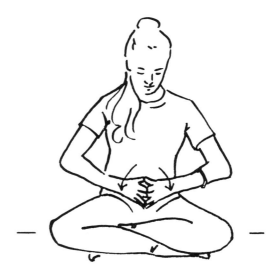

Adjustments, Hips, Thighs, and Legs
(about 12 min)

1. Lie down on your back, arms at your sides. Spread your legs wide and bring them 18 inches from the floor. Bring your right foot to your left thigh as you inhale deeply. Then exhale completely as you extend your right leg back out, at the same time bringing the left foot to the right thigh. Continue this wide-leg bicycling motion *for 1-3 min.*

2. Sit up, legs spread wide. Grab your left foot or ankle with both hands and gently bounce up and down *20 times*, inhaling as you go up and exhaling as you go down. Then switch legs and gently bounce *another 20 times.*

3. Still sitting up, legs spread wide, grab one big toe with each hand, thumb pressing into the fleshy underside of the toe throughout the exercise. Inhale as you bring your body up, straight spine, to center **(a)**, then exhale as you bring your head to your left knee **(b)**. Inhale bringing your body up to center **(a)**, then exhale as you bring your head to your right knee **(c)**. Do this 4-part exercise *a total of 20 times.*

4. Now sit on your left heel, right leg stretched out in front of you. Grab your right big toe with your right hand and your right heel with your left hand. Inhale, making the spine as straight as possible **(a)**, then exhale as you bring your head down to your right knee **(b)**. Do this a total of *20 times.* Then switch legs and do it *20 more times.*

5. Come into rock pose and place your palms flat on the floor a few inches in front of your knees. In this position, inhale completely as you flex your spine forward **(a)**. Then exhale as you flex your spine back **(b)**. Continue this modified spine flex *for 3 min.* Then inhale, exhale, and relax.

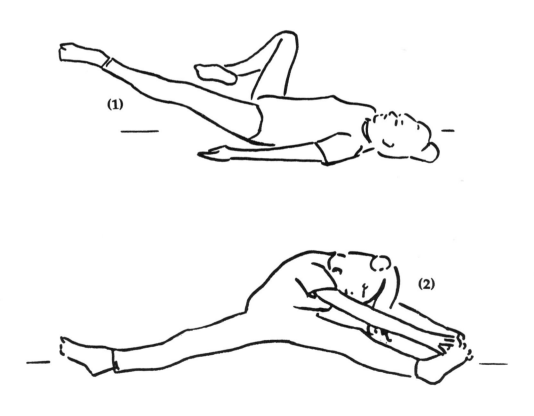

(1)

(2)

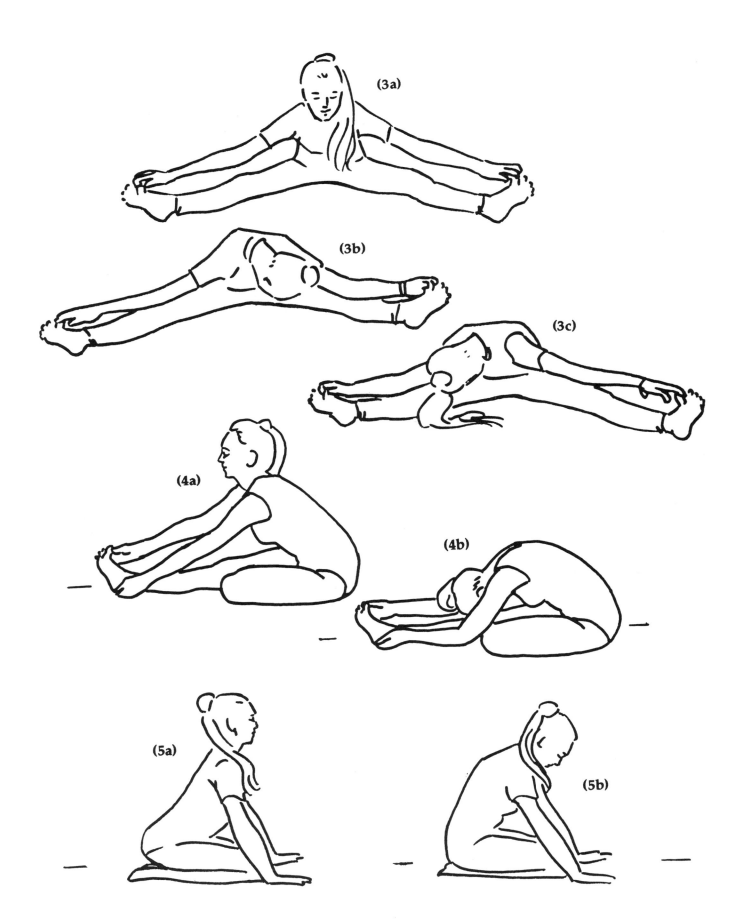

(3a)

(3b)

(3c)

(4a)

(4b)

(5a)

(5b)

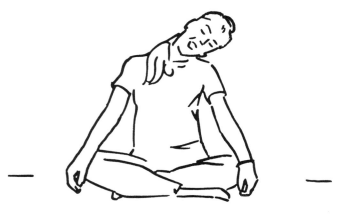

Adjustments, Jaw
(2 min)

Sit in easy pose. Open the mouth as wide as possible. Bend the neck and place the head on the left shoulder. Then place it on the right shoulder.

Continue this movement *for 2 min.*

Adjustments, Knees—see "Adjustments, Ankles and Knees"

Adjustments, Legs—see "Adjustments, Hips, Thighs, and Legs"

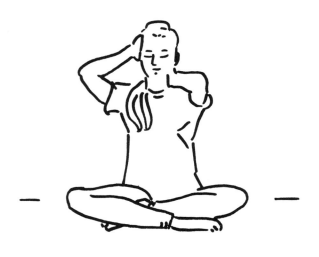

Adjustments, Neck
(4-6 min)

Sit in easy pose. Place the palm of the left hand on the left rear of the neck. Place the palm of the right hand above the right ear with the fingers extending to the back of the head. Look at the tip of the nose. Push in with maximum pressure with both hands.

Continue for 2-3 min, then reverse the position for 2-3 min. The breathing will become heavy.

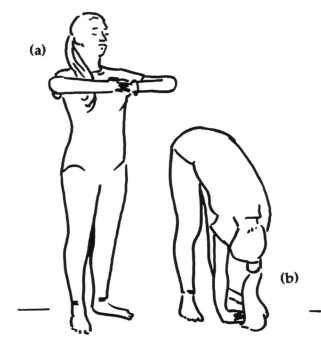

(a)

(b)

Adjustments, Pelvis
(about 2 min)

Stand with the feet slightly spread, palms down, hands in open Venus lock at the level of the armpits **(a)**. Bend forward from the hips, bringing the hands down toward the floor, hands still in Venus lock, with no bend in the legs **(b)**.

Rhythm: Take 1 second to lower yourself and 1 second to rise up. *Continue for 52 cycles.*

For a pelvic adjustment set, see **Keeping Up with Kundalini Yoga,** pp. 28-29.

Adjustments, Spine
(8 min)

Stand up, hands in prayer pose. Raise the left leg and place the sole of the foot on the inside of the right thigh so the heel touches the groin **(1a)**. This is **tree pose.** *Continue for 2 min.*

Now bring the palms together overhead. Totally stretch the arms up, keeping the elbows straight **(1b).** *Continue for 2 min.*

Switch legs and repeat both parts of the exercise *for 2 min each.*

Comments
The heel of the raised foot rests on the pelvic bone. The body is balanced, with the spine firm. In this position, there is pressure at the base of the spine; all the vertebrae are automatically adjusted. Generally, women more than men have this capacity to adjust themselves. This exercise is also good for women with **menstrual problems.**

For a set dealing with self-adjustment of the spine, see **Slim and Trim: Exercises and Meditations for Women,** pp. 22-23.

Adjustments, Thighs—see "Adjustments, Hips, Thighs, and Legs"

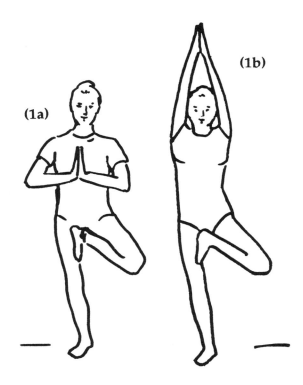

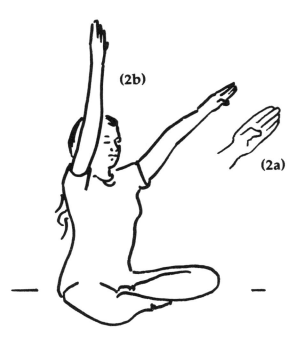

Adrenal Gland Imbalance
(11 min)

Sit in easy pose. Make sure the spine is pulled up and stretched straight. Extend the right arm straight up hugging the ear. Extend the left arm to 60° from horizontal, with the palm facing down. On both hands, put the thumb onto the mound just below the little finger **(2a).** Keep the eyes slightly open. Look down toward the upper lip. Press the elbows straight. Stretch the arms up from the shoulders **(2b).**

No breath is specified; however, the breath will automatically become longer and deeper as you continue. It is important to hold the arms perfectly still at the angles given, with a stretching feeling in the shoulders, to receive the full benefit. *Continue for 11 min.*

Comments
This meditation is a direct healer for the **kidneys** and **adrenal glands.** Consequently, it helps repair the energy drained by long-term **stress.** It alleviates problems of the **lower spine,** and helps the **heart.** Be sure to allow yourself at least as much time afterwards to relax as it took you to do the exercise.

See also "Heart Attacks, to Prevent."

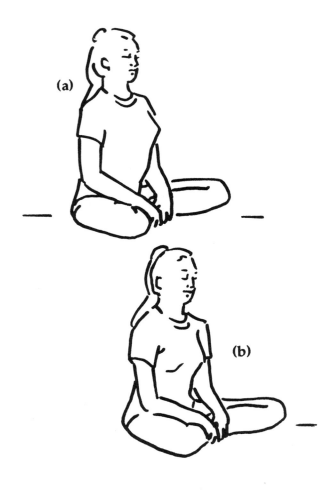

Aging
(about 3 min)

Spine flex: Grab the ankles with both hands and deeply inhale. Flex the spine forward and lift the chest up **(a)**. As you exhale, flex the spine backwards **(b)**. Keep the head level so it does not flip-flop. *Repeat 108 times,* then relax.

Comments

Aging does not start with years; it begins with nutritional deficiency, intestinal problems, and an inflexible spine that disrupts the flow of spinal fluid. In fact, in India age is measured by the flexibility of the spine.

A study done at the University of California, Davis, in 1973 showed that this spinal flex exercise, besides limbering up the spine, created a multistage reaction pattern that greatly altered the proportions and strengths of alpha, theta, and delta waves in the brain. You may notice that you feel calmer and more centered after doing it.

See also "Blood Disease"; "Youthfulness, to Regain"; **Sadhana Guidelines,** pp. 45-46 and 47-50; and **Keeping Up with Kundalini Yoga,** pp. 10-13.

Alcohol—see "Addiction"

Ankles, Stiff
(4 min)

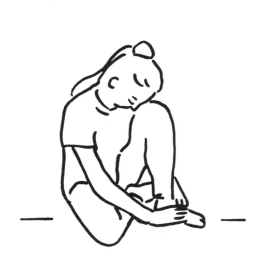

Sit in a comfortable position with the left foot on the floor within reach of the hands. Massage the Achilles tendon with the thumbs of both hands. The area to rub is from the heel up the tendon about 4 inches. If you press correctly, the toes will flex slightly. Rub firmly and rhythmically *for 2 min.*

Switch legs, and rub *for another 2 min.*

Comments

Rubbing near the heels breaks up long-term calcium deposits or "crystals."

Arteries, to Flush—see "Tennis Elbow"

Arthritis
(1-3 min)

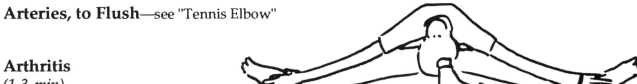

Sit down with legs spread as wide apart as possible. Catch your heels. Touch your forehead to the floor. Make sure the legs stay straight. Breath is normal. *Continue for 1-3 min.*

Comments
This exercise is also good for **constipation** and **eyesight.** See also "Leukemia."

Cold showers are excellent for arthritis. Don't precede or end your cold shower with warm water. See also **Foods for Health and Healing,** pp. 99-100.

Asthma
(1-3 min)

Stand up, heels together. Hands are overhead with palms together. Lean back as far as possible and do breath of fire *for 1-3 min.* To avoid falling, stand over a gymnast's horse or a soft sofa back or get someone to stand behind you to catch you if you lose your balance. You must bend back as far as possible.

Comments
This exercise is said to make asthma fly away like a crow at the clap of your hands!

Back, Lower, Pain—see "Abdomen, Weak"

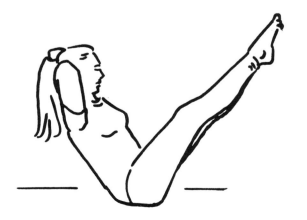

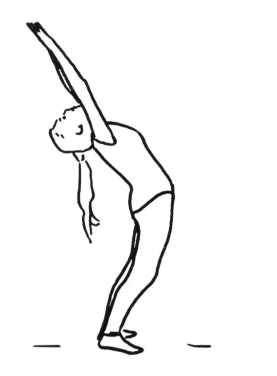

Back, Morning Pain
(3-10 min)

Lie on your back. Lock your hands in Venus lock under the neck, touching the skin of the neck (under your hair, if it's down). Slowly raise the legs and torso to 60°. Hold this position as long as possible, anywhere between *3 and 10 min.* Focus on your feet and let the breath come naturally.

Comments
This is a hard one! Mentally repeat a mantra, such as SAT (as you inhale) and NAAM (as you exhale) to help you through it.

This exercise is also good for **balance,** and for resetting the magnetic field on waking up.

For a set of exercises dealing with lower back pain, see **Keeping Up with Kundalini Yoga,** pp. 28-29.

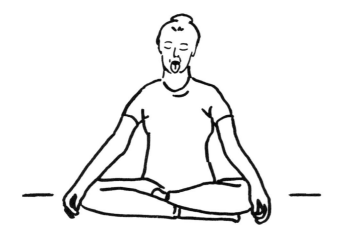

Back, Pain in Small of—see "Colon, to Cleanse"

Bad Breath, Chronic
(time variable, once a day for 15 days)

Sit in easy pose. Stick out your tongue. Breathe through the mouth until the tongue tastes bitter, as if it had quinine on it. Do this practice *once a day for 15 days.*

Balance—see "Back, Morning Pain"

Bladder, Weak—see "Excretory System, to Improve"

Blood, to Cleanse
(11 min)

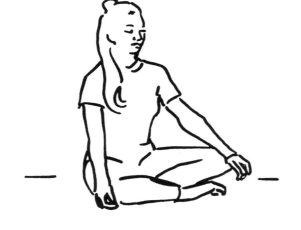

Sitting in easy pose, inhale deeply and chant in one breath RAA RAA RAA RAA, MAA MAA MAA MAA, SAA TAA NAA MAA (*aa*'s as in "far"; see musical staff below). Hands can be in gyan mudra. *Continue for 11 min.*

Comments
This "Charity of Breath Meditation" is very cleansing to the bloodstream. The rate of breathing slows down from about 15 breaths/min to about 8 breaths/min, lending calmness and clarity to the mind as well.

See also "Blood Disease"; "Circulation, to Improve"; "Heart Attacks, to Prevent"; "Leukemia"; and "Tennis Elbow."

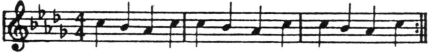

RAA RAA RAA RAA MAA MAA MAA MAA SAA TAA NAA MAA

Blood Cells, to Balance Red and White
(11 min/day for 40 days)

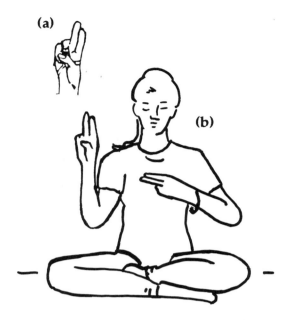

Sit in easy pose with a straight spine. With the right elbow bent and relaxed near the body, raise the right hand up to the side as if taking an oath. Middle and index fingers of the right hand are pointed up, other two fingers curled down under the thumb **(a)**.

Hold the left hand in the same mudra, with the two outstretched fingers touching the heart center, midway between the nipples. Make the outstretched fingers as straight as possible. Eyes are either closed or focused on the tip of the nose **(b)**. Breathe slowly, meditatively, and with control, taking the breath mentally from the nose up to the third-eye point and then down to the heart where the fingers are.

Continue for 11 min. Then inhale and exhale deeply 3 times, and relax.

Comments

This meditation helps balance the distribution of the white and red blood cells. This balance is intimately involved in the proper functioning of the body's **immune system.** Do the meditation once a day for 40 days in order to perfect it.

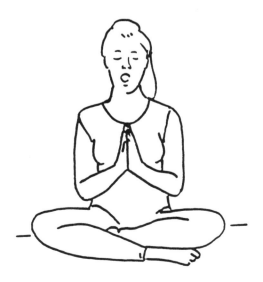

Blood Disease
(18 min, 1 hour, or 108 breaths)

Sit with a straight spine, palms touching at the chest, arms hugging the ribs. Focus on the tip of your nose. Mouth is open. Inhale in 4 equal strokes, mentally concentrating on one syllable of the mantra WAA-HE GU-ROO with each stroke, and on the breath as it crosses the tongue tip. Exhale in 4 equal strokes, concentrating on each syllable of the mantra WAA-HE GU-ROO, and on the breath as it crosses the tongue tip.

Continue for 5 min. Then rest for a minute.
Repeat all the above twice.

Comments

Anyone who can practice this kriya an hour a day is greatly strengthened against diseases of the blood. Doing the breath described in this kriya 108 times **purifies and oxygenates the blood.** Doing it as described above for 18 min a day for 40 days will **rejuvenate an old body.**

Blood Pressure, High
(1-3 min or 40 min)

Sit in easy pose. Use the thumb of the right hand to block the right nostril. Fingers of the right hand are together, pointed straight up. Do breath of fire through the left nostril while pumping the navel point in and out **(1a)**. The more completely you can pull your abdomen in and push it out, the more effective will be the kriya. *Continue for 1-3 min.*

For longstanding problems of high blood pressure, do *40 min daily* of normal left nostril breathing (without breath of fire or stomach pumping).

Comments
Breath through the left nostril stimulates the cooling, relaxing functions in the body. The breath flows mainly through only one nostril at any one time. The flow of breath, which switches from one nostril to the other every 2 1/2 hours throughout the day, can be automatically channeled to the left nostril by holding the left hand under the right armpit, with the right arm pressing in on it slightly in its normal relaxed position **(1b)**. Try it!

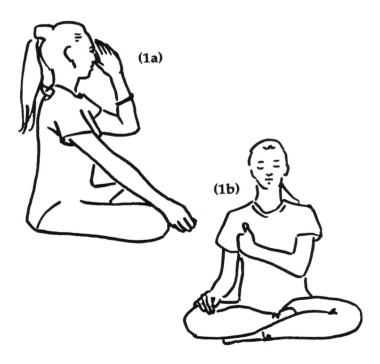

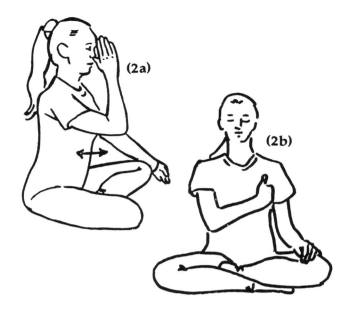

Blood Pressure, Low
(1-3 min or 40 min)

Sit in easy pose. Use the thumb of the left hand to block the left nostril. Fingers of the left hand are together, pointing straight up. Do breath of fire through the right nostril while pumping the navel point forcefully in and out **(2a)**. *Continue for 1-3 min.*

For longstanding problems of low blood pressure, do *40 min daily* of normal right nostril breathing (no breath of fire or stomach pumping).

Comments
Breath through the right nostril stimulates the "sun" functions of the body—when you have a lot of sun energy you do not get cold easily; you are energetic, extroverted, and enthusiastic. It is the energy of purification. It holds the weight down. It aids digestion. It makes the mind clear, analytical, and action-oriented. The breath flows mainly through only one nostril at any one time. The flow of breath, which switches from one nostril to the other at regular intervals during the day, can be automatically channeled to the right nostril by holding the right hand under the left armpit, with the left arm pressing in on it slightly in a normal, relaxed position **(2b)**.

Boils—see "Colon, to Cleanse"

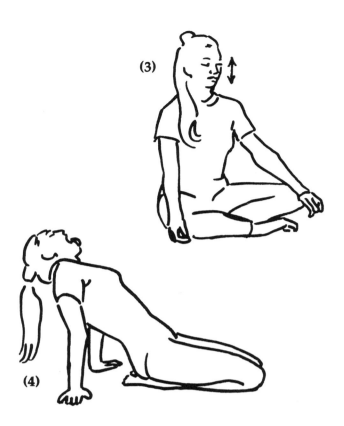

(3)

(4)

Brain, to Rejuvenate
(8-9 min)

Sit in easy pose with your hands on your knees. Hold your chest out and shoulders back. Begin vibrating the front of your face using very rapid, short up-and-down vibrating motions **(3)**. Try to move just the forehead. The breath will adjust itself. *Continue for 8-9 min.*

Comments
Mastak Subhaee Kriya changes and replaces the grey matter in the brain.

Calcium–Magnesium Imbalance
(about 5 min)

Sit in rock pose. Place the hands on the floor behind the body and arch up into half camel pose. Open the mouth wide and stick out the tongue **(4)**. Inhale completely; as you exhale, laugh down deep in your belly **("belly laugh")**. *Do a total of 10 of these* inhaling–exhaling–laughing cycles. Then relax on your back *for 3 min.*

Cancer, Breast, Prevention
(5-6 min)

Lie down on your stomach. Bend one leg toward your head and grasp the ankle with both hands. Arch the body up **(one-leg bow pose) (5a)**. Rock back and forth on the abdomen, exhaling as you go forward and inhaling as you go back. *Continue for 1 min.*

Switch legs and repeat the process for another minute. Then grab your left ankle with your left hand and your right ankle with your right hand, arch up in **regular bow pose (5b)**, and rock back and forth *for 1 min.* At the end of the exercise, inhale completely, exhale completely, pull root lock on the held exhalation, and then relax completely for a few minutes on your stomach, head turned to the left.

Comments
Exercises that flush the chest area help prevent breast cancer. See also "Tennis Elbow." See **Foods for Health and Healing** for foods that help fight cancer.

A good, hard set of exercises recommended for women to help prevent cancer, **menstrual problems,** and excess **emotionality** can be found in the **Yoga Manual,** pp. 30-34.

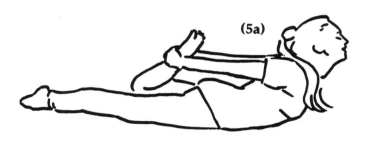

(5a)

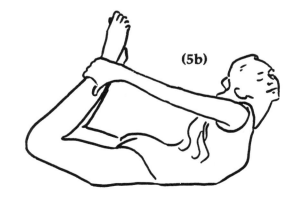

(5b)

Cataracts
(about 5 min)

Sit down with your legs together on the floor in front of you. Place your palms on the floor behind you and lean back to 60° from the floor. Drop your head back and fix your eyesight on a point on the ceiling **(1a).** Don't wink or blink. Do breath of fire *for 2 min.* Then inhale and raise both feet 12 inches from the floor, keeping the vision steady **(1b).**

Hold for 15-20 seconds, then exhale down. Repeat the breath of fire *for 1 min.* Inhale and raise both feet 12 inches. *Hold for 15 seconds.* Exhale down and relax completely on the back.

Comments

This exercise, which energizes the brain and eyes, is helpful in cases of eye disease such as cataract and for **headaches.**

Chest Mucus—see "Coughing"

Cholesterol—see "Circulation, to Improve"

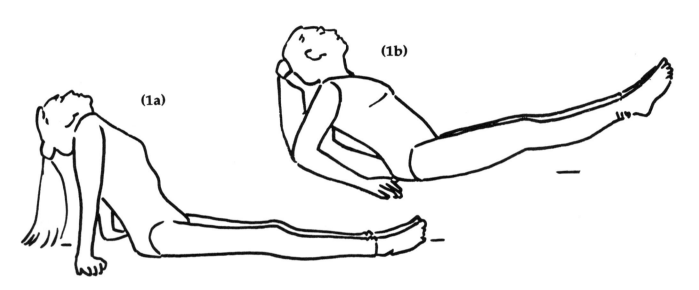

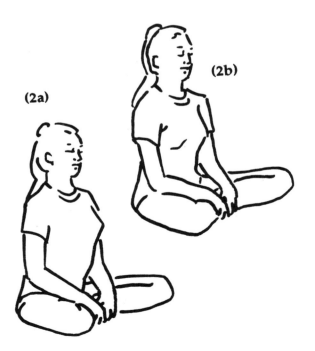

Circulation, to Improve
(1-3 min)

Sit in easy pose and grasp your ankles. Inhale completely. Exhale and pump your abdomen in and up **(2a),** then out **(2b)** on the held exhalation. Continue pumping until you must inhale; then inhale, exhale, and begin pumping again. *Continue for 1-3 min.*

Comments

This kriya **cleans the blood,** removes **cholesterol,** and improves circulation in the capillaries. See also "Heart Problems" and "Tennis Elbow."

For sets of exercises to improve the circulation, see the **Sadhana Guidelines,** pp. 65-66 and 85-86, and **Slim and Trim,** pp. 20-21.

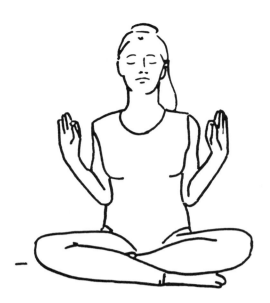

Cocaine Habit, to Break
(8-9 min)

Sit with arms bent up and to the sides, hands in gyan mudra. Press the shoulder blades together hard. Eyes are closed.

1. Inhale, and hold the breath in *for 1 min.* Exhale. *Repeat twice.*

2. Relax, breathing normally, *for 2-3 min.*

3. Get back into the posture. Inhale, and press the tongue with all your strength against the roof of your mouth. Apply root lock *for 30 seconds.* Exhale. Do breath of fire *for 15-20 seconds. Repeat.*

4. Inhale. Press the tongue against the roof of the mouth *for 1 min.* Exhale and relax.

Comments

This kriya balances the **nervous system** and acts as a check on the **parasympathetic nervous system**. It helps break the cocaine habit and alleviates withdrawal symptoms. It is an especially good kriya for women.

Colds

Most colds and flu come from an energy imbalance that starts in the digestive tract. See "Digestion, to Improve."

Colon, to Cleanse
(3 min)

Sit in rock pose. Cross your hands over your navel **(a).** Lower your forehead to the floor. Swing the buttocks back and forth like a pendulum **(b).** *Continue for 3 min.*

Comments

Walking a mile a day greatly improves elimination. For sets of exercises to improve elimination, see the **Meditation Manual,** pp. 14-16; **Slim and Trim,** pp. 14-15; and **Sadhana Guidelines,** pp. 52 and 55-56.

This kriya is also helpful for **pain in the small of the back,** and for **pimples, rashes,** and **boils.**

Complexion—see "Thyroid Gland Imbalance"

Constipation—see "Arthritis." See also **Foods for Health and Healing,** pp. 93-94.

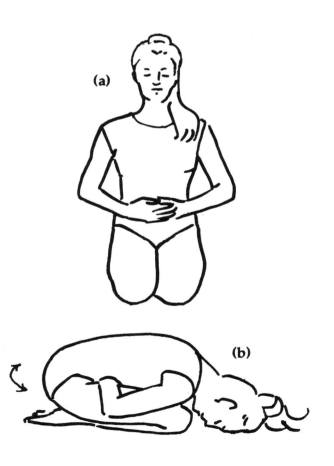

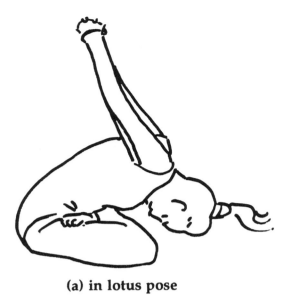

(a) in lotus pose

Coughing
(2 min)

Sit in lotus pose, or rock pose if lotus is too difficult. Clasp the hands in Venus lock behind your back. Bend down till your forehead touches the floor and stretch the locked hands up as far as possible above your back in **yoga mudra (a, b).** Feel at peace. *Continue for 2 min.*

Comments
This pose helps alleviate coughing and dissipate mucus in the chest. Do for *2 min once an hour* while ill.

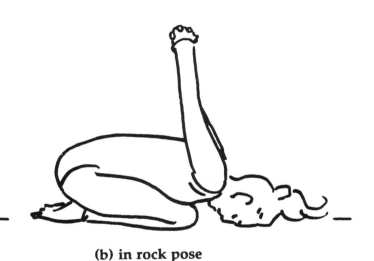

(b) in rock pose

Deafness, to Prevent
(10 min)

Get into rock pose. From this position, raise the buttocks and lower your head until one ear is resting on the floor. The pressure of your upper body weight should be on that ear. Rest in this position *for 5 min*, then switch ears and continue *for 5 more min.*

Comments
Practiced regularly, this kriya helps prevent deafness.

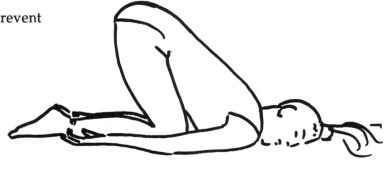

Depression

(3-11 min)

Sit with a straight spine in easy pose. Arms are extended straight out in front of you, parallel to the floor. Close your right hand into a fist. Wrap the fingers of your left hand around your right-hand fist. The bases of the palms touch. The thumbs are close together and are pulled straight up. The eyes are focused on the thumbs.

Now inhale *for 5 seconds* (do not hold the breath in); exhale *for 5 seconds;* hold the breath out *for 15 seconds*. Continue.

Start with 3-5 min and work up to 11 min. Build up the time slowly. In time, you can work up to holding the breath out for 1 full minute. However, take care not to hold the breath out so long as to make yourself dizzy or nauseous.

Comments

This meditation is an antidote to depression. You will find that, properly done, it totally recharges you. It will give you the capacity to deal well with life. See also "Heart Problems."

Other meditations against depression can be found in the **Sadhana Guidelines,** p. 106, and in the **Survival Kit,** pp. 12, 28, and 30.

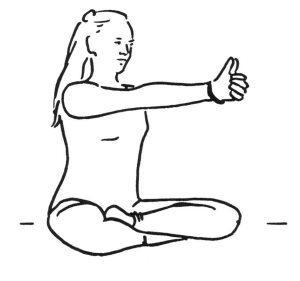

Diabetes Mellitus

(1-3 min)

Sit in easy pose. Inhale completely. Exhale completely, and hold the air out as you pump the navel in and up **(1a)**, then out **(1b)**, again and again. Continue on the held exhalation *for 15-60 seconds*. When you need to take a breath, inhale, exhale, and begin pumping again on the held exhalation. Continue this practice *for 1-3 min*.

Comments

This technique takes sugar out of the bloodstream. It is not recommended for hypoglycemics.

Other techniques that help alleviate diabetes mellitus are beak breath (the mouth is pursed in a tight "o" like a beak and the breath inhaled either in one long stroke or in short sips) *for 31 min* **(1c)**, maha mudra *for 15 min* **(1d)**, and foot massage at the pancreas point **(1e)**.

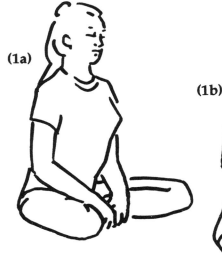

(1a)

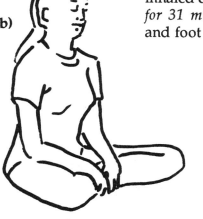

(1b)

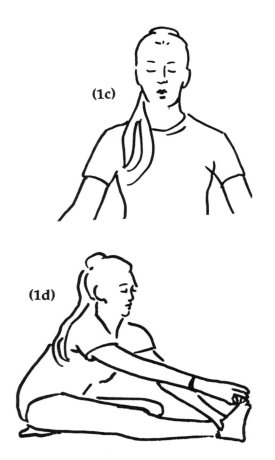

(1c)

(1d)

pancreas point

(1e)

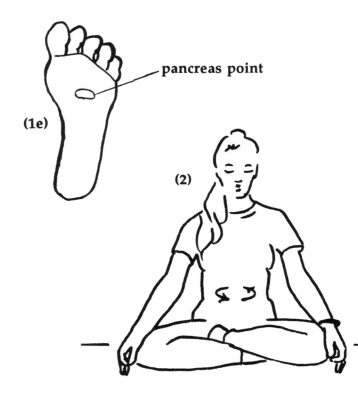

(2)

Digestion, to Improve
(a minute or so)

This **Vatsar Dhouti Kriya** should only be done on an empty stomach, and never more than twice a day. If you are doing other exercises as well, make this the last exercise in the series.

Sit in easy pose, hands on the knees. Apply neck lock. Make a beak of the mouth and drink in air through the beak. Hold the air in as long as possible as you churn your stomach round and round **(2)**. When you must exhale, do so through the mouth **without pressure.** *Do the exercise a total of 3 times at one sitting.* **Then drink 2 quarts of water, and avoid hot, spicy foods for the rest of the day.**

Comments

For digestive problems when your stomach is full, see "Digestive Problems, Emergency." Vatsar Dhouti Kriya is said to eliminate all digestive problems, including chronic excess acidity. Since many other diseases, such as **colds** and **flu,** start with problems of digestion and elimination, the kriya works toward general health as well.

See also "Lymph Glands, to Improve." Sat kriya (Appendix A) is also good for the digestion. For sets of exercises for the digestive tract, see the **Meditation Manual,** p. 17, and **Sadhana Guidelines,** pp. 52 and 59.

Notes on Digestion: You cannot digest your food properly unless you schedule relaxation into your days. (This doesn't mean more sleep!) You also need mild daily activity, such as walking a mile or so, to keep your body strong and healthy, and to massage the organs of digestion and elimination. During the day, take a 10-min nap after eating. In the evening, take a walk after your meal. This will stimulate your digestive system so that when you sleep, your body can be totally at rest, not diverting energy to the digestive process.

Digestive Problems, Emergency
(15 min)

This kriya requires a fair amount of spinal flexibility. Kneel in rock pose. Lower yourself until your body is supported by the elbows and the back of the head (modified **fish pose**) **(3)**. Begin breath of fire *for 15 min.*

Comments
This kriya is for emergency digestive problems such as overeating and stomach pain. Take extra care in getting into and out of this posture, so as not to wrench a muscle.

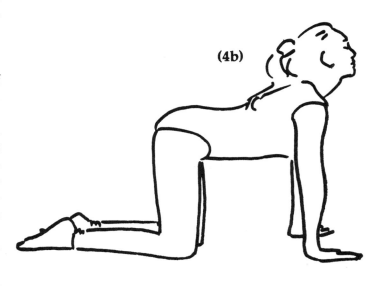

(3)

Drug Damage to Nerves
(3 min/day for 40 days)

Get onto your hands and knees. Begin flexing the spine up **(4a)** and down **(4b)**, inhaling as the spine goes down, and exhaling as it goes up (**cat–cow pose**). The neck is arched back on the inhale. *Continue for 3 min.*

Comments
To repair nerve damage due to misuse of drugs, do this exercise *once a day for 40 days.* Also, drink "golden milk" daily during this time. To make golden milk, boil 1/8 teaspoon turmeric in 1/4 cup water for about 8 min, till it forms a thick paste. If too much water boils away, add a little more. Meanwhile, combine 8 ounces of milk with 2 tablespoons of raw almond oil and bring to a boil. As soon as the mixture begins to boil, remove it from the heat. Combine the two mixtures and add honey to taste.

(4b)

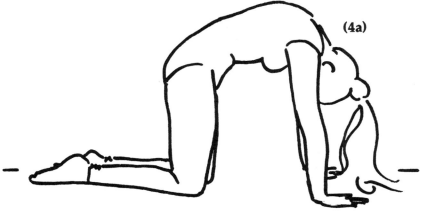

(4a)

Drug Dependence—see "Addiction"; "Cocaine Habit, to Break"; "Heroin Convulsions"; "Marijuana Brain."

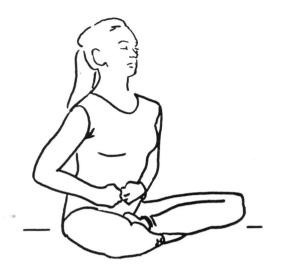

Dysentery, Chronic
(10-15 min)

Sit in easy pose, hands in fists at the navel point. Inhale completely. Exhale completely, and press the fists into the navel area on the held exhalation. When you can no longer hold the breath out, inhale, exhale, and begin pressing again. *Continue for 10-15 min.*

Comments
See also **Foods for Health and Healing**, pp. 33, 37, 94.

Ears, to Cleanse
(6 min)

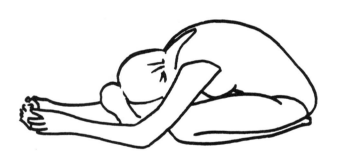

Sit on the left heel, the right leg stretched straight forward in front of you. Grabbing your extended toes or ankle with both hands, put the left ear on the right leg, or as close to it as you can get it. Hold the position while doing breath of fire *for 3 min.* Then switch legs and ears and repeat *for 3 min.*

Comments
This **Kanar Kriya** can also be done in half lotus.

Elimination, to Improve—see "Colon, to Cleanse"

Emotional Balance
(10 min)

Sit in easy pose, left hand in gyan mudra and resting on the left knee. Bring the right hand up to nose level, fingers together and pointed up. Use the thumb to close the right nostril as you inhale deeply through the left nostril **(a)**. Then use your little finger to block the left nostril as you exhale deeply through the right nostril **(b)**. Continue this deep, alternate-nostril breathing *for 10 min.*

Comments
If you feel emotional, drinking several glasses of water will help restore balance. A women's meditation for emotional balance can be found in **Slim and Trim,** p. 24. The sets of exercises on pp. 30-34 of the **Yoga Manual** and on p. 61 of the **Survival Kit** also help overcome emotionality.

Epilepsy
(up to 31 min)

Sit on your left heel, right leg over the left, left foot flat on the floor, in **hero pose.** The hands are cupped, little fingers touching along their length, in front of the chest as if you were about to receive an offering. Chant like this continuously:

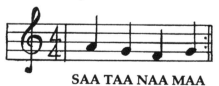

SAA TAA NAA MAA

Continue for up to 31 min. (3 min and 11 min are two good stopping places.)

Comments
This meditation is helpful in cases of epilepsy and for **headaches.**

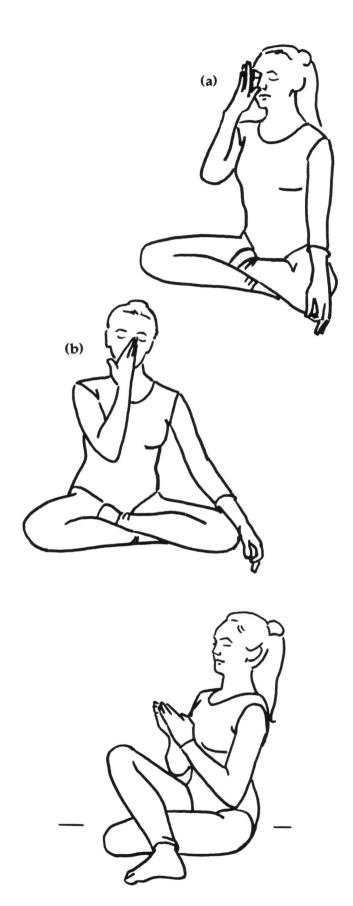

65

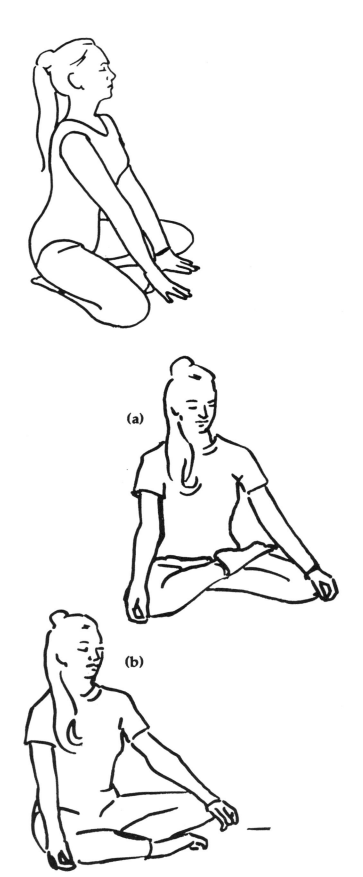

(a)

(b)

Excretory System, to Improve
(3-4 min)

Sit on your heels, knees wide, toes together. Fingertips are on the floor, elbows straight, arms perpendicular to the floor. Lift the body up slightly, supporting its weight on your fingertips. Inhale completely. Exhale, hold the breath out, and pump the navel point in and out *5 times* on the held exhalation. *Relax for 1 min.* Then inhale completely, hold the breath in, and pump *15 times.* Exhale completely and pump *15 times* on the held exhalation. *Then relax for 1 min.*

Comments
Good for the **kidneys** and **bladder.** This is a moderately hard, very effective kriya. Be sure to follow directions carefully.

Eye Pain
(up to 31 min)

Sit in lotus pose **(a)**, or in easy pose **(b)** if lotus pose is too difficult. Hands are resting on the knees in gyan mudra. Apply neck lock. Concentrate at the third-eye point. Roll the tongue back in your mouth and suck on it. Begin long, deep breathing. As you inhale, pull root lock and mentally visualize the sound SAT rising along the spine. Think NAAM out the top of the head as you exhale.

Continue for up to 31 min (3 and 11 min are also good stopping places).

Comments
Called **"Maha Karma Shambhavi Kriya,"** this meditation is considered good for alleviating pain in the eyes, and for coordinating the energy of the optic nerve. It has many other benefits as well: It purifies and opens the chakras, helps one gain control of the breath, helps eliminate **irritations of the body,** and allows one to "harness the 3 powers of God" (generating, organizing, and destroying).

Eyesight, to Improve
(6-11 min)

Sit in easy pose, head and neck straight. Place palms together in prayer pose, fingers pointing up, forearms at chest level and parallel to the floor. Without bending your neck, look with both eyes at your thumbs. Do long, deep breathing *for 6-11 min.*

Comments
Regular practice of this kriya improves eyesight and helps prevent eye trouble. See also "Arthritis" and "Tennis Elbow." For sets to improve eyesight, see the **Meditation Manual,** pp. 39 (**vision correction**) and 40 (**myopia**). More information on eyes is available with the **Tratakam Meditation Photo** (see Appendix C).

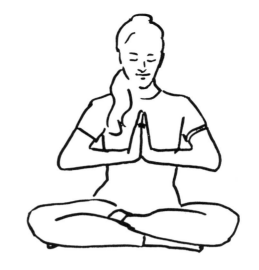

Fatigue, General—see "Mental Fatigue"

Fever
(minimum of 3 min)

Sit in easy pose, hands in gyan mudra at the knees **(a).** Roll the tongue into a "U," with the tip just outside the lips **(b).** Inhale deeply through the rolled tongue; exhale through the nose. *Continue for a minimum of 3 min.*

Comments
This exercise, known as **Sitali Kriya,** is well known for its ability to lower fevers, bring **blood pressure** to normal, and cure **digestive ailments.** It is said to impart **power, strength,** and **vitality.** At first the tongue will taste bitter as toxins are expelled, then it will become

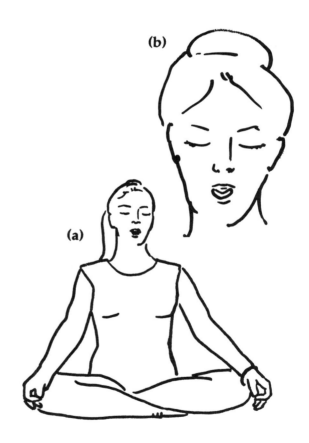

sweet. This is a sign of improved health.

Sitali Kriya is an excellent breath to practice *26 times in the morning and 26 times in the evening every day.*

Flu

Most colds and flu come from an energy imbalance that starts in the digestive tract. Please see "Digestion, to Improve."

Gallbladder Problems
(2-6 min)

Lie on your back. Place the right hand under the small of the back, palm down. Place the left palm against the back of the neck, elbow touching the floor. Raise the right leg to 90° **(a)**. Do breath of fire *for 1-3 min*. Then inhale completely, hold the breath in *for about 15 seconds*, exhale, and relax down into corpse pose **(b)**. Deeply relax in this position *for 1-3 min*.

Comments
This kriya is useful in correcting problems of the gallbladder, **heart,** and **spleen.**

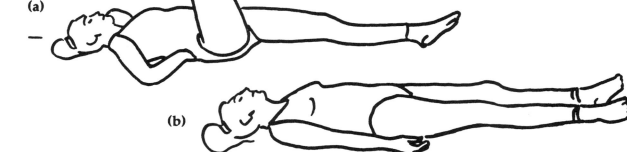

(a)

(b)

Gas, in Men
(1-3 min)

Lie down on your back. Bring the knees tight to your chest, clasping the hands round the knees. Raise your head and tuck your nose between your knees. Do breath of fire *for 1-3 min*.

Comments
Besides alleviating gas in men, regular practice of this exercise stimulates the **thyroid gland** and frees up the **sacral area** of the back.

Gas, in Women
(1-2 min)

Sit down, right leg extended straight out in front of the body. Place the left foot on top of the right thigh. Place the hands in Venus lock behind the back. Bring the head to the knees and raise the hands as high as possible. Relax in this position *for 1-2 min.*

Comments
This kriya is good for the **ovaries,** for **regulating menstruation,** and to alleviate gas in women.

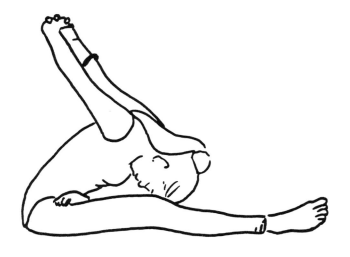

Glandular System, to Balance
(3-5 min)

Sit in easy pose with a straight spine. With the elbows bent, raise the hands up and in until they meet at the level of the heart a few inches from the body. With the fingers of both hands extended and joined and the palms toward the body, place the palm of the right hand over the back of the left hand. The fingers of the left hand point to your right, and the fingers of the right hand point to your left.

Press the tips of the thumbs together. Hold the hands and forearms parallel to the floor. Eyes are 9/10 closed. Inhale deeply and hold the breath in *for 10 seconds.* Exhale completely and hold the breath out *for 10 seconds.* (The air must go completely out on the exhalation; this will trigger a state of alarm in the brain and central nervous system for a few seconds.) Concentrate powerfully on the breath. *Continue for 3-5 min.*

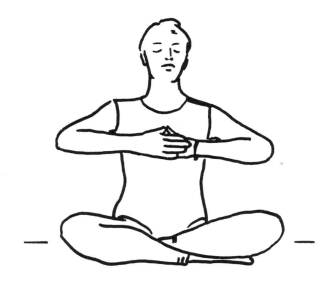

Comments
This meditation brings both the **nervous** and the **glandular system** into balance in a matter of minutes. See also "Heart Problems." For sets of exercises for glandular balance, see the **Sadhana Guidelines,** p. 72; **Slim and Trim,** p. 19; and all the sets in **Maintenance Yoga.**

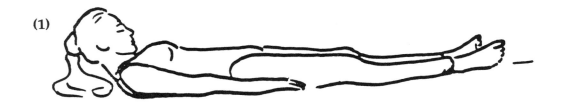

(1)

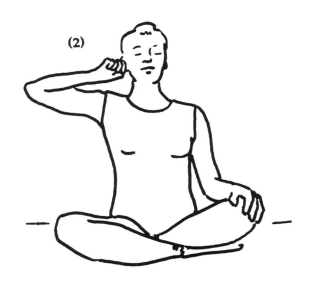

(2)

Hearing, to Improve—see "Tennis Elbow"

Heart—see "Gallbladder Problems"; "Sympathetic Nervous System, to Repair"; and "Tennis Elbow"

Heart, to Relax
(1-5 min)

Sit in easy pose, left hand resting on the left knee. Grasp your right ear with your right thumb and forefinger, right elbow pulled back **(2)**. Relax the left side of the body as you rigidly tense the right side of the body. Battle both to relax the left and to tense the right! *Continue for 1-5 min.*

Heart Attacks, to Prevent
(7-31 min)

With a straight spine, sit with the left heel at the perineum (the area midway between the genitals and the anus). The right knee is at the chest, right foot flat on the floor. Forearms are parallel to the floor, right palm resting on top of the left hand. Both hands are flat; tips of thumbs are touching. Eyes are only 1/5 open. Look down as deeply as possible **(3)**.

Completely inhale in 4 equal sniffs. Exhale completely in 4 equal parts. (This is called **broken breath**.) You may use any mantra you wish with the breath. A good one is ONG ONG ONG ONG repeated mentally as you inhale and SOHUNG SOHUNG SOHUNG SOHUNG repeated mentally as you exhale.

Continue for 7 min. Adding 5 min for each week of practice, you may work up to 31 min per session.

Grey Hair—see "Youthfulness, to Regain"

Headaches
(1-3 min)

Lie down on your back. Raise your head off the floor and do long, deep breathing *for 1-3 min* **(1)**.

Comments
Also see the entries "Cataracts," "Epilepsy," and "Migraine."

70

Comments

According to yogic theory, the ida, pingala, and sushumna are the three most important nerve currents in the body. The 4-fold breath indicated in the above exercise stimulates the center where these nerve currents meet. It assists in absorption of oxygen into the **lungs** and **purifies the blood.** As the exhalation is 25-30% greater than usual, old toxins are forced out into the bloodstream.

The pressure of the right knee on the liver helps balance the energy of the liver and **spleen.** The mudra stimulates and regulates the interaction of the **pancreas, adrenals,** and **kidneys.** Stimulation of the perineum balances the **sexual glands.**

Regular practice of this kriya helps prevent heart attacks. It is a very powerful aid to longer life.

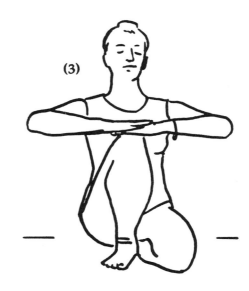

(3)

Heart Problems
(11-31 min)

Sit in easy pose with a straight spine. Place the palms gently together with the fingers extended and joined and the thumbs crossed. With the elbows straight, extend the arms 60° up and as far to the left as possible. The fingertips of the right hand cover the mounds at the base of the fingers of the left hand. Be sure to keep the elbows stretched out and up and locked throughout the meditation **(4).**

Inhale powerfully and deeply through the nose. Exhale powerfully through the mouth, pushing the navel deeply in toward the spine. Concentrate on the breath.

Continue for 11 min. (You can build up to 31 min with practice.) At the end of the meditation, inhale deeply, exhale very powerfully and completely, hold the air out for 10-15 seconds, then relax.

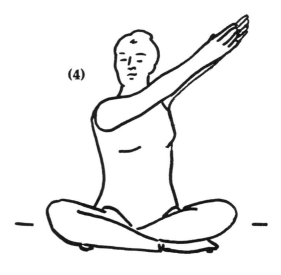

(4)

Comments

This meditation is good for people who have any kind of heart problem, **tension,** or **poor circulation.** It is also good for the **glandular system** and for **depression.** Various meridians in the shoulders and elbows will ache as the body corrects itself, but keep the elbows locked regardless! If you've been eating junk food you may find it hurts more; you will feel very weak no matter how strong you may be!

For sets of exercises to strengthen the heart, see **Sadhana Guidelines,** pp. 51 and 65.

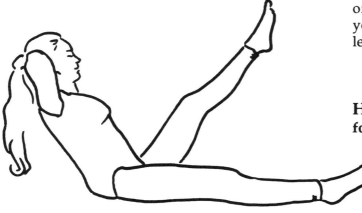

Heart Valves, to Strengthen
(1-3 min)

Sit down with the feet stretched out in front of you, hands clasped in Venus lock behind your head. Lean back to 60° and bring your left leg up to 60°.

Maintain this position *for 1-3 min*.

Hemorrhoids–see "Urethritis." See also **Foods for Health and Healing,** pp. 94-95.

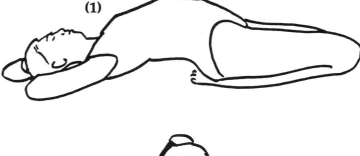

(1)

Hepatitis
(28 min)

1. Sitting on your heels, hands in venus lock on the neck (underneath the hair), rest your back on the floor. Do breath of fire *for 2 min.* Inhale, hold the breath in *for 10-15 seconds,* then relax.

2. Sitting on your left foot, place your right foot on your left thigh. Fingers of the right hand are on the ground; the left hand is in gyan mudra, resting on the right foot. Do breath of fire *for 2 min,* then inhale, exhale, and relax.

3. Stand stooped over, hands in venus lock at crotch level. Do breath of fire through the mouth *for 2 min.* Inhale, hold the breath in *for 10-15 seconds,* then relax.

4. Sit in easy pose, arms straight out to the sides parallel to the ground, palms down. As you do breath of fire, rock from side to side on the buttocks, keeping the arms parallel to the ground. Continue *for 2 min,* then inhale and relax.

5. Sit in easy pose with the left foot on the right thigh. Grab the left toe with both hands, and do breath of fire *for 2 min.*

6. Sit on the left heel with the right leg straight forward. Lean back on your hands and arch up high, head back. Do breath of fire *for 2 min.*

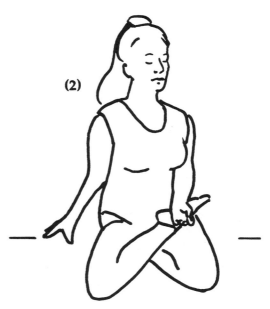

(2)

7. Sit with your legs straight forward. Grab your toes. Inhale, exhale, pull root lock, and pump the stomach in and out until you can no longer hold the breath out. Inhale, exhale, and pull root lock. *Repeat this step.*

8. Completely relax.

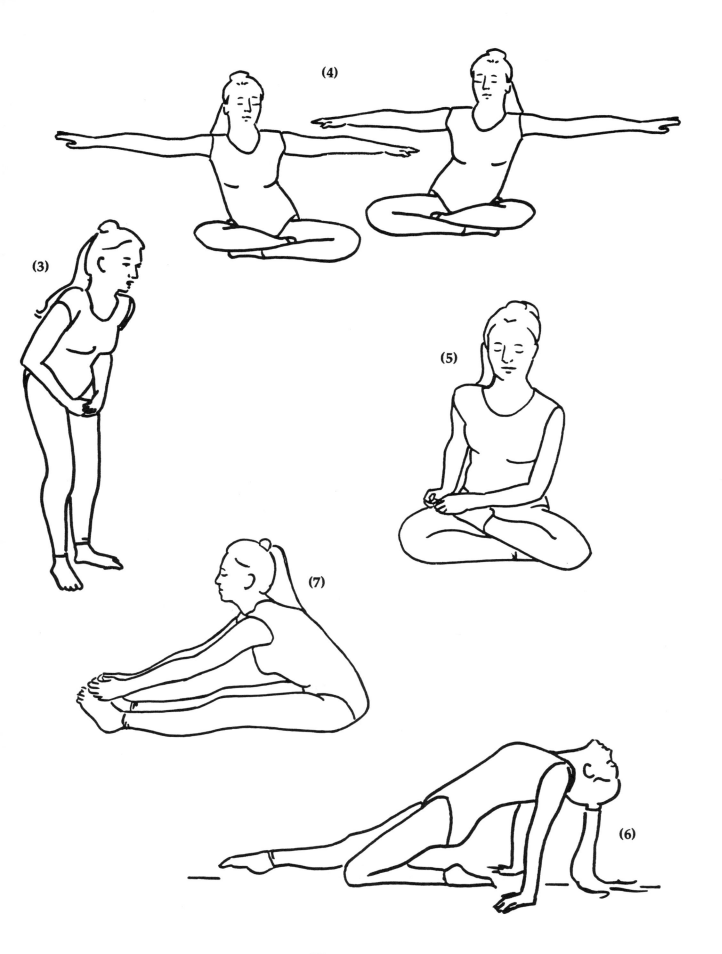

(4)

(3)

(5)

(7)

(6)

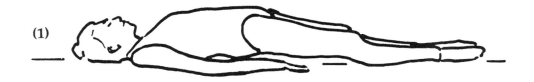

(1)

Hernias, to Prevent
(1-3 min)

Lie down on your back. Raise only the hips off the floor. Hold this position *for 1-3 min* **(1).**

Heroin Convulsions
(at least 33 min)

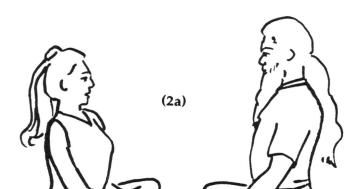

(2a)

Sit facing a friend, each of you in easy pose, hands holding your ankles, and begin flexing your spine back and forth (spine flex). Look into your friend's eyes and chant SAT as the spine flexes forward **(2a),** NAAM as it collapses backward **(2b).**
Continue for 30 min.

Comments
Drink raw onion juice once an hour for a few hours, then once every 3 hours. Rub your palms and the soles of your feet with raw onion juice once or twice daily for 7 days.

Do not work on the navel point. When you do the chant, breathe deeply; inhale deeply between each repetition. If you are helping a friend through heroin convulsions, look directly into their eyes during the exercise and encourage them to breathe deeply throughout.

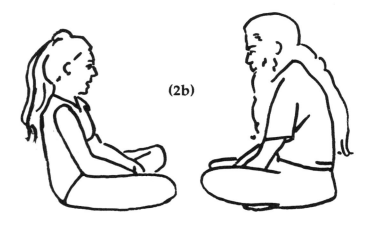

(2b)

Hypoglycemia
(1 1/2 min)

Lie down on your stomach. Grab your ankles and arch up into bow pose. Bend your neck to touch left ear to left shoulder **(3).** Hold this position *for 45 seconds.* Then change so that the right ear touches the right shoulder. Hold *for another 45 seconds.*

Comments

See also "Ileocecal Valve, to Unblock." Pulling diaphragm lock is also helpful in cases of hypoglycemia. For dietary hints, see **Foods for Health and Healing,** pp. 84, 91.

Ileocecal Valve, to Unblock
(2-3 min)

Sit in rock pose or easy pose. Massage yourself under the armpits *for a few minutes* **(4).** If the ileocecal valve is jammed, this will help free it. The meridian stimulated also improves the **pancreas** and helps treat **hypoglycemia.**

Immune System, to Bolster—see "Blood Cells, to Balance Red and White"

Indigestion—see "Digestion, to Improve" and "Digestive Problems, Emergency"

Insanity
(3-31 min)

Sit in easy pose with a straight spine. Relax the arms and hands in any meditative posture. Focus on the tip of the nose. Open the mouth as wide as possible **(5a).** Touch the tongue to the upper palate **(5b).** Breathe normally **through the nose.** *Start with 3-5 min of practice*, building with time to 11 and then 31 min, if desired.

Comments

This meditation gives immediate relief to any wavering, spaced-out mind. If psychiatric help is not available, try this meditation. Practicing the kriya allows one to still the most restless mind.

See also "Menstrual Irregularity after Birth Control Pills"; "Mental Fatigue." Less dramatic meditations for mental balance can be found in the **Survival Kit,** pp. 34-38. A meditation for ego problems and mental disease can be found in **Keeping Up with Kundalini Yoga,** p. 30.

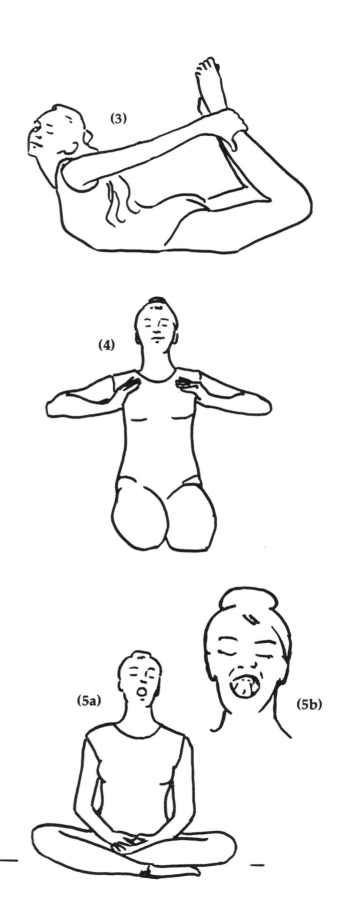

Insomnia
(6-21 min)

Lie down on your back. From this position, get up on all fours **(bridge pose),** keeping the middle body in a straight line **(1a).** Let the head relax back. Do breath of fire *for 5-20 min.* Then inhale completely, hold the breath *for about 15 seconds,* exhale, and relax down onto your back.

Inhale completely, reaching with open hands up towards the ceiling **(1b).** Hold the breath in, make fists of the hands, and very slowly, with isometric tension so great as to make the hands and arms shake, bring the fists down to the chest **(1c).** When they reach the chest **(1d),** exhale and relax.

Comments
For a set of exercises dealing with sleep difficulties in general, see **Sadhana Guidelines,** pp. 77-78.

Intestines, to Cleanse—see "Colon, to Cleanse"

Irritations of the Body—see "Eye Pain"

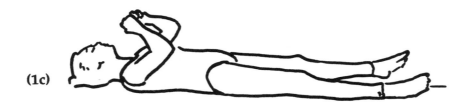

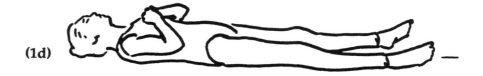

(1a)

(1b)

(1c)

(1d)

Kidneys
(1-3 min)

Place your right foot on your left thigh. Place your left knee next to the chest, foot flat on the floor. Bring your left arm straight up in the air, hand in gyan mudra. Place your right arm behind your back, palm on the floor behind you. Raise your body up and balance on your right palm and left foot as you do breath of fire **(2)**. *Continue for 1-3 min.*

Comments
Drinking 2 quarts of water daily just after getting up is very beneficial to the kidneys. See also "Adrenal Gland Imbalance"; "Excretory System, to Improve"; "Heart Attacks, to Prevent"; and "Menopause."

Knee Trouble, to Prevent
(6 min)

Stand with legs straight and feet slightly apart. Cross your arms over your chest, hands on opposite arms just above the elbows **(3a)**. Maintaining your balance with care, lift your right foot slightly **(3b)**, then lift the right leg across the left leg until the right heel meets the left side of the left knee **(3c)**. Next, bring your right foot back to slightly off the floor **(3b)**. Finally, bring the weight back onto both feet. The entire 4-count cycle should take about 4 seconds.

Continue with the right foot *for 3 min,* then switch to the left foot and continue *for 3 more min.*

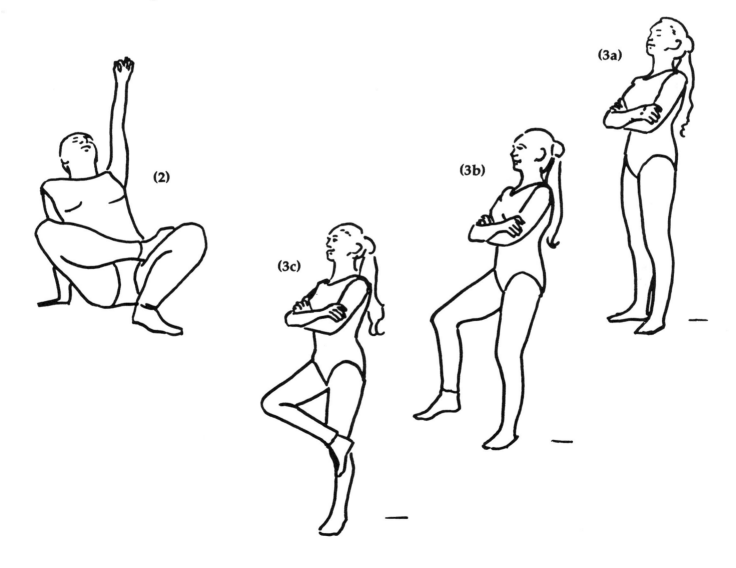

(2)

(3a)

(3b)

(3c)

Leukemia
(a little over 2 1/2 hours)

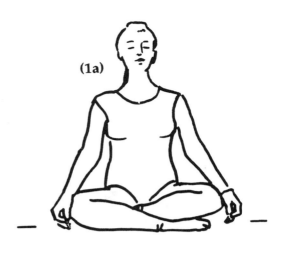

(1a)

Sit in easy pose with your hands in gyan mudra **(1a)**. Eyes are closed and pressed up toward the third-eye point. Inhale completely in either 3, 4, or 5 parts **(broken breath)**. As you exhale, chant out loud WAAHE GUROO, WAAHE GUROO, WAAHE WAAHE WAAHE GUROO.

Continue for 2 1/2 hours.

Now sit in easy pose with your left hand behind and at the middle of your back, palm outward at the level of your heart. The right palm is on your chest, in the middle, at heart level **(1b)**. Chant:

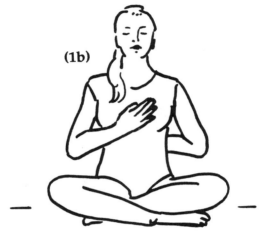

(1b)

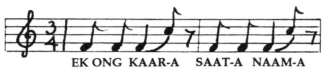

EK ONG KAAR-A   SAAT-A NAAM-A

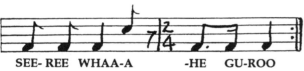

SEE- REE WHAA-A   -HE   GU-ROO

The navel point is pulled in sharply on EK. On each high-pitched *a* sound (pronounced like *u* in "bus") the diaphragm is pulled up so that the rib cage lifts. On -HE the diaphragm and stomach relax. Low-pitched *aa*'s are pronounced as in "far." Other vowel sounds are as follows: *e* as in "gate," *o* as in "hope," *ee* as in "see," *u* as in "good," and *oo* as in "mood."

As you chant, visualize the energy spinning from the base of the spine upward through the top of the head to infinity. *Continue for 3 or 11 min.*

Comments
This meditation is helpful in cases of leukemia, **arthritis,** and **to cleanse the blood.**

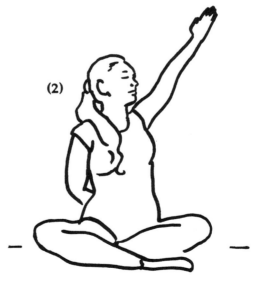

(2)

Liver, to Cleanse
(1-3 min)

Sit in easy pose, the right arm behind your back, left arm up at 60°, fingers stretched straight up, elbow straight **(2)**. Maintain the posture as you swing left and right *for 1-3 min.*

Comments
Do not use this exercise in cases of severe liver disorder. See also "Heart Attacks, to Prevent," and "Menopause."

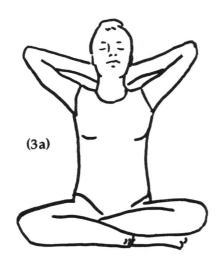

(3a)

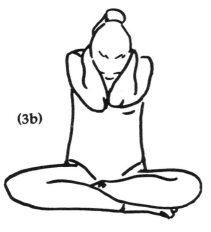

(3b)

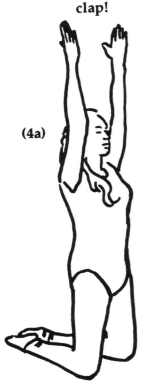

clap!

(4a)

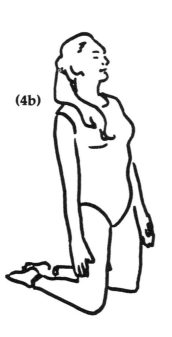

(4b)

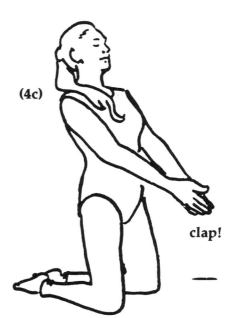

(4c)

clap!

Lung Capacity, to Expand
(1-3 min)

Sitting in easy pose, place your hands in Venus lock on the back of the neck (under your hair, if it's down). Inhale deeply, bringing the elbows up and back, head erect **(3a)**. Exhale completely as you bring your chin to your chest and your elbows down and close in to your sides **(3b)**. *Continue for 1-3 min.*

Comments
See also "Heart Attacks, to Prevent." For a set of exercises to expand the lung capacity, see **Sadhana Guidelines,** p. 80.

Lung Problems, to Prevent
(1 min)

Kneel up on the knees, head facing forward. Inhale, raise the hands up over the head, and clap them together 1 time **(4a)**. Exhale, dropping the hands to the sides of the body **(4b)**. Swing the arms loosely forward, clapping the hands again **(4c)**. Then raise the arms overhead, inhaling and clapping as the 3-phase exercise begins again: clap, drop, clap; clap, drop, clap. *Continue for 1 min.*

Comments
For a set of exercises to strengthen the lungs, see **Sadhana Guidelines,** pp. 85-86.

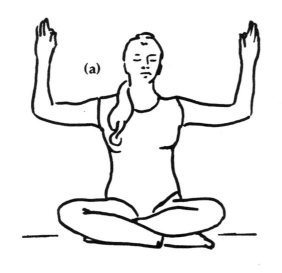

(a)

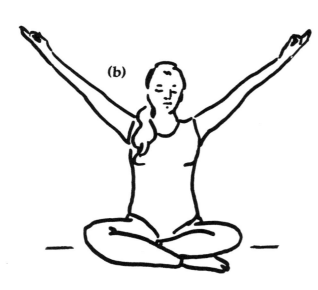

(b)

Lungs, Impurities in Upper
(1-3 min)

Sit in easy pose, hands in gyan mudra, upper arms out from the shoulders to either side parallel to the floor, forearms pointed straight up toward the ceiling **(a)**. Inhale completely and raise the arms up toward the ceiling **(b)**. Exhale completely and lower them to the original position. Continue at a rapid pace *for 1-3 min.*

Lymph Glands, to Improve
(2 min for each of 3 independent exercises)

1. Sit down with your legs extended wide in front of you. Sit with spine erect and hands on top of the knees. Inhale deeply as you flex the spine forward **(1a)**. Exhale deeply as you flex the spine back **(1b)**. Keep the knees straight throughout. *Continue for 2 min.*

2. In the same position, place palms flat on the floor about 18 inches in front of the groin. Keep the spine straight. Put as much pressure as possible on the palms and heels, as if you were trying to lift yourself off the floor. Keep the tension while doing long, deep breathing *for 2 min.*

3. Sit in easy pose. Make both hands into fists. Extend the arms out straight alternately in a punching motion, inhaling as the arms pass each other and exhaling as each arm reaches its full extension. The breath will become breath of fire. *Continue for 2 min.*

Comments
These exercises are not a set. Each of them may be done separately. The first two drain the **lymph glands from the groin and thigh** areas. The last one removes toxins from the **lymph glands of the shoulder area;** it is also good for the **digestion.**

For a longer set of exercises to cleanse the lymph system, see **Maintenance Yoga,** pp. 11-14.

Lymph System—see "Tennis Elbow"

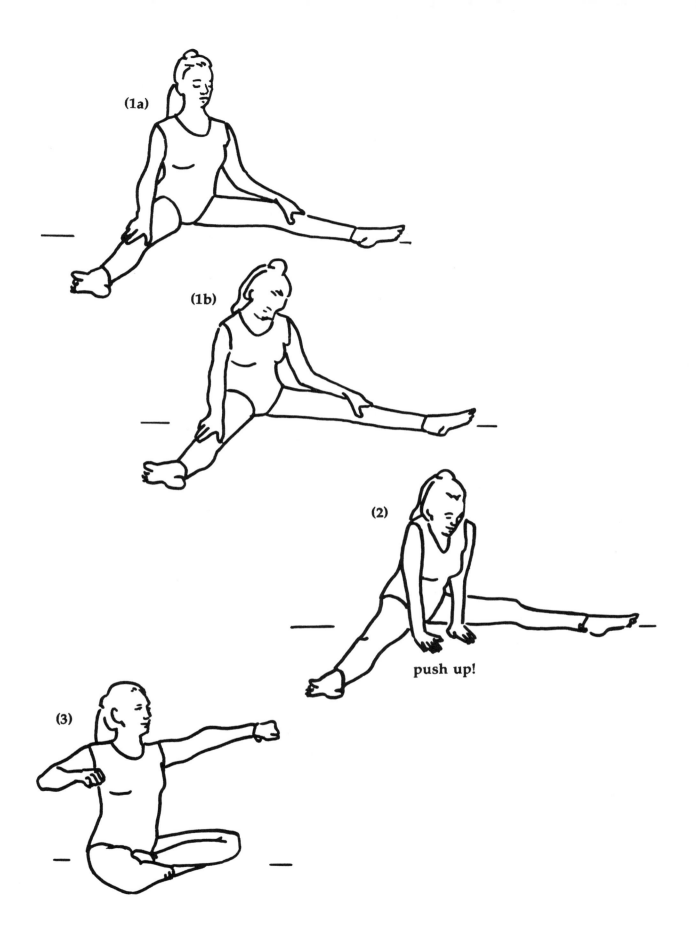

(1a)

(1b)

(2)

push up!

(3)

81

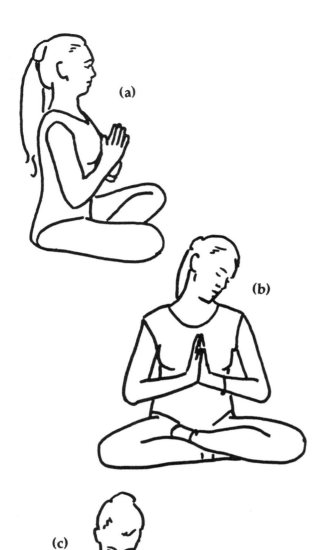

Marijuana Brain
(11-31 or 60 min)

Maha Agni Pranayam: Sit in easy pose or lotus pose. Apply neck lock. Place the palms flat together 9-12 inches in front of the chest at heart level **(a)**. Inhale completely and swing the head from the right shoulder **(b)** across the chest **(c)** to the left shoulder **(d)**. Complete the swing by pulling the chin in (neck lock) while facing straight forward **(a)**. Now focus at the third-eye point and project this mantra silently in perfect rhythm:

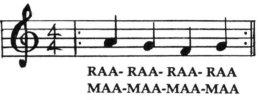

RAA- RAA- RAA- RAA
MAA-MAA-MAA-MAA
RAA- RAA- RAA- RAA
MAA-MAA-MAA-MAA
SAA - TAA -NAA -MAA

Exhale and immediately swing the head again as you inhale. The head swing should be quick and should give a little pull at the base of the skull. *Continue for 11 min.* You can build up to 31 min at a sitting with practice.

Comments

The term "pothead" derives from a state of mind peculiar to those who use marijuana. This state of mind is said to be caused by blockage of spinal fluid and acupressure meridians at the base of the neck. The meditation above eliminates this neck block. It can also help your desires to become aligned with what you achieve through action.

Note: On the fourth and eleventh days of the moon cycle, there is a special pressure on the endocrine system to cleanse itself. You may thus find it particularly effective to practice this meditation *for 1 full hour* on either of these special days.

Menopause
(11 min maximum)

Sit on your right heel and extend your left leg straight behind you with no bend in the knee. Let the head fall back so the spine is arched as much as possible. Bend the arms with the elbows as close to the sides as possible, hands at shoulder height with palms toward the ceiling. Hold the position *for 5 min* with long, deep breathing. Then switch sides and continue *for 5 more min* (a total of 11 min maximum).

Comments
This exercise is a great help for women going through menopause, and also to prepare for this stage of life. It also helps keep the **ovaries, kidneys,** and **liver** healthy.

See also "Premenstrual Syndrome, for Prevention and Alleviation."

Menstrual Pain
(3 min for each independent exercise)

1. Lie down on your stomach. Place your palms on the floor next to your shoulders and, keeping your feet together and arms straight, arch up into **cobra pose**. Hips should stay on the floor. Arch the neck back and look up at a point on the ceiling **(see next page)**. Hold the pose with long, deep breathing *for up to 3 min*. Then relax on your stomach.

2. Lie down on your stomach. Take hold of your ankles and pull yourself up into bow pose. Again, arch your head back. Hold the position with long, deep breathing *for up to 3 min*. Then slowly come down and relax.

3. Lie down on your back. Bring your heels together and raise your legs 45°, keeping the legs straight. Relax into the pose *for up to 3 min* with long, deep breathing.

4. Lie down on your stomach. Make fists under the abdomen, above the hip joint. Keeping the chin on the floor, heels together and legs straight, raise just your legs as high as you can. Hold for *up to 3 min* with long, deep breathing, then relax.

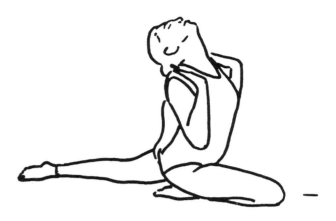

Comments
These 4 exercises are not a set. Any of them may be done individually to help relieve menstrual pain. Be careful not to do them with breath of fire or any very powerful breathing.

To prevent menstrual pain altogether, be certain that you are getting ample calcium in your diet. Massage your ovaries every morning. Do breath of fire *(3 min)* and **stretch pose** (lie on your back, raise your head and heels 6 inches from the floor, and do breath of fire) *for 3 min* **(5)** at least once a day except when having your period. This will keep your navel point centered. (When the navel point is displaced, a woman cannot achieve orgasm.)

The navel point can be displaced particularly easily by the following means during menstruation:
- carrying heavy objects,
- carrying objects on one side of the body,
- exposure to cold water (don't swim),
- doing too much work, and
- not relaxing.

See also "Adjustments, Spine"; "Premenstrual Syndrome, for Prevention and Alleviation." For a set of exercises dealing with menstrual problems, see the **Yoga Manual**, pp. 30-34. For more information on the navel point, see the **Meditation Manual**, pp. 5-13.

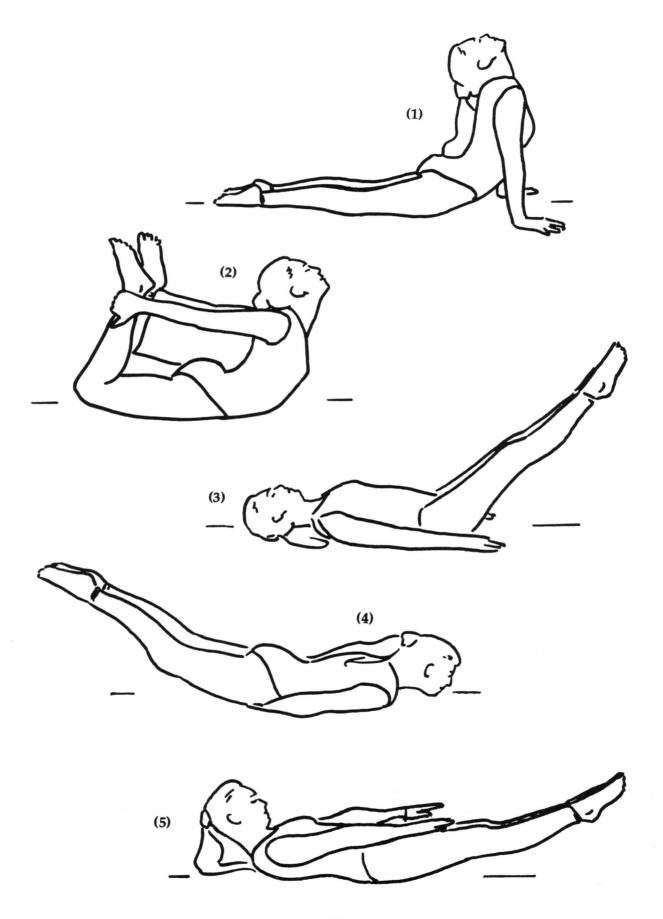

Menstrual Regularity
(30 min)

Sit in easy pose with hands resting on the knees **(a).** You will be meditating on the mantra SAA TAA NAA MAA to the following melody:

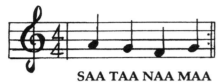

SAA TAA NAA MAA

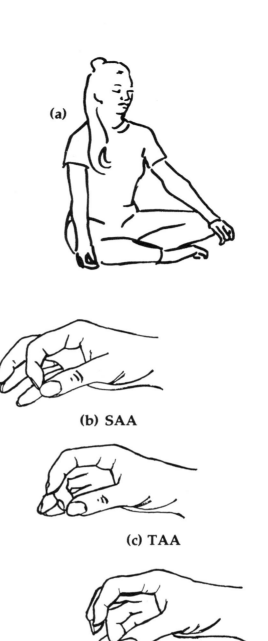

(a)

On SAA, touch the first finger of each hand to the corresponding thumb **(b).** On TAA, touch the middle finger to the thumb **(c).** On NAA, touch the ring finger to the thumb **(d).** On MAA, touch the little finger to the thumb **(e).** The chanting takes place in a cycle: a normal voice, a strong whisper, and silently.

Begin in a normal voice *for 5 min,* then whisper *for 5 min,* then go deep into the sound silently *for 10 min.* Then come back to the whisper *(5 min),* and then to the normal voice *(5 min).*

When you have finished, inhale completely, then exhale all the air out. Stretch the hands up as far as possible and spread them wide. Stretch the spine up and take several deep breaths. Then relax.

Note: To avoid getting headaches while practicing this meditation, visualize with each syllable of the chant that energy is flowing in through the top of your head and, proceeding along an L-shaped path, out your third-eye point **(f).**

(b) SAA

(c) TAA

(d) NAA

(e) MAA

Comments

This **Kirtan Kriya** will help your body re-establish a menstrual rhythm after discontinuing use of birth control pills. It also brings a very stable sense of **mental balance.**

See also "Gas, in Women."

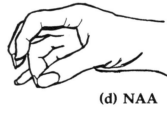

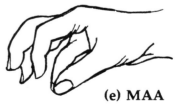

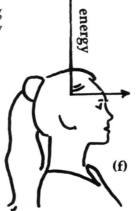

energy

(f)

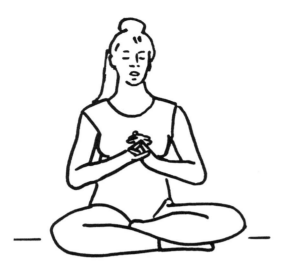

Mental Fatigue
(3 min)

Sit in a comfortable, meditative posture, spine straight. Place your ring fingers together and interlace all the other fingers, right thumb on the top. Hold your hands several inches out from your diaphragm with the ring fingers pointed upwards at a 60° angle.

Close your eyes. Inhale deeply and powerfully. Exhale as you chant out loud the mantra ONG ("ooonnnnnnnnnnnnnng"). Keep your mouth open, but let all the air flow through your nose as you chant. The sound is far back and up in the soft palate.

Continue for 3 min.

The power of this chant, when correctly done, must be experienced to be believed. Only *5 repetitions* are necessary to totally elevate the consciousness.

Comments

This meditation should only be done when you can relax afterwards. Done correctly, it is very effective against "brain drain," imparts a **balanced mental state,** and can give you **absolutely powerful energy.**

For a set of exercises dealing with mental fatigue, see the **Yoga Manual,** pp. 20-23.

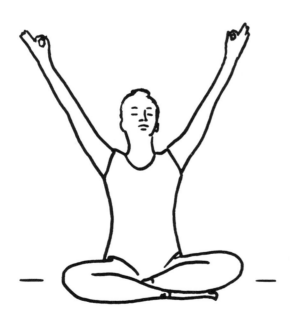

Migraine
(12 min minimum)

Sit in easy pose, hands in gyan mudra, arms straight at a 70° angle out and up from the sides. With closed eyes, look to your hairline. Hold the posture with normal breathing *for at least 11 min.* Then relax the hands down onto the knees and chant, in a monotone, "We are the love" *for 1-2 min.*

Comments

This meditation is good for **headaches,** especially migraine. Pain in the back and behind the shoulders while doing it is a sign of weak blood circulation.

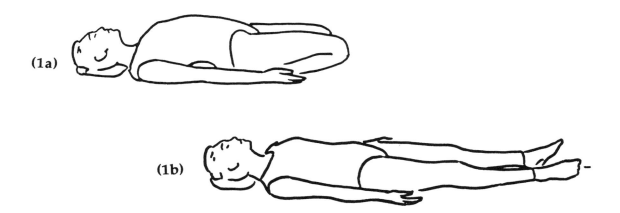

(1a)

(1b)

Mineral Imbalance
(2-4 min)

This exercise requires a fair degree of body flexibility. Sit on the heels. Carefully lean back so that the shoulders touch the floor. Rest the hands next to the thighs **(1a)**. Do powerful breath of fire for *1-3 min*. Then inhale, hold the breath in briefly *(about 15 seconds)*, exhale, and deeply relax on the back, legs stretched out **(1b),** *for 1 min.*

Comments

This exercise promotes mineral balance in the body by regulating the glands. The deep relaxation at the end of the exercise allows the glandular secretions to be circulated and distributed throughout the body.

Muscles, to Regenerate—see "Youthfulness, to Regain"

Nerves, to Balance
(1-3 min)

Lie down on your back, left arm along your side. Raise the right arm and left leg, toe pointed, to 90° **(2)**. Hold the position *for 1-3 min.*

Comments

See also "Cocaine Habit, to Break." Meditations and sets of exercises for balancing the nervous system can be found in the **Survival Kit** (pp. 23, 56-58) and the **Sadhana Guidelines** (pp. 61-62, 67-68, 105). See also "Glandular System, to Balance."

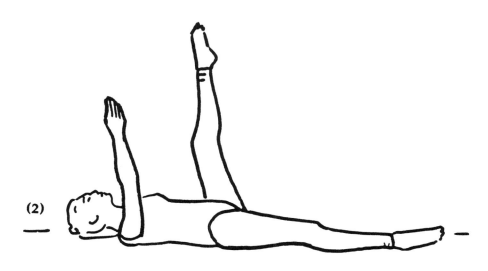

(2)

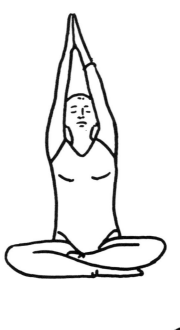

Nerves, Weak
(3 min)

Sit in easy pose. Bring the arms up straight, hugging the ears, palms together overhead. Do long, deep breathing *for 3 min.*

Comments

Another meditation for strong nerves can be found in the **Survival Kit,** p. 36.

Nervous System, Diseases of
(1-3 min)

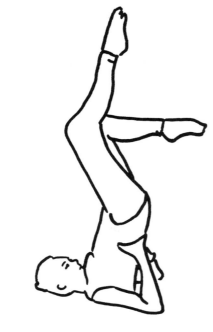

Lie down on your back. Bring your body up into **shoulder stand,** supporting the back with the hands. Make the body as straight as possible throughout the exercise. Begin kicking the buttocks sharply with alternate heels. As one heel kicks, the other is straight up in the air. *Continue for 1-3 min.*

Comments

This exercise is helpful in conjunction with traditional treatment of diseases of the nervous system. See also "Cocaine Habit, to Break."

Ovaries, to Relax
(1-3 min)

Lie down on your back. Take hold of your ankles and draw your heels to your buttocks, with the heels about 18 inches apart. Raise your entire torso up off the floor, arching the spine, as if pressing the navel point to the ceiling. Hold this position *for 1-3 min.* Then slowly come down, stretch out the legs, and relax.

Comments

This exercise is good for problems of the ovaries, and for tension in them. It also strengthens the **sciatic nerves.**

See also "Gas, in Women" and "Menopause."

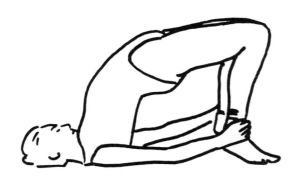

Overeating–see "Addiction"; "Digestive Problems, Emergency"

Pancreas, to Strengthen
(6 min)

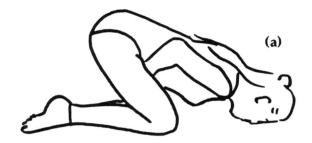

Kneel in rock pose, hands crossed over your navel. Bring your forehead to the floor and your buttocks up to 60° **(a)**. Maintain the position *for 3 min.*

Still kneeling in rock pose, hands on the knees, lean back 60° from the floor **(b)**. Maintain the position *for 3 min.*

Comments
See also "Heart Attacks, to Prevent"; "Ileocecal Valve, to Unblock."

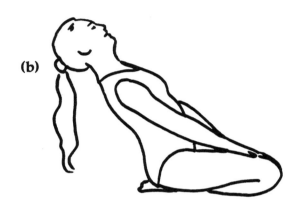

Parasympathetic Nervous System—see
"Cocaine Habit, to Break"

Parathyroid Gland Imbalance
(up to 11 min)

Crouch down on your right leg, left leg trailing behind you like a tail. The left knee is off the floor. The hands are at the chest, palms together. Focus on the tip of your nose. As you inhale, mentally say the sound RAA (*aa* as in "far"). As you exhale, mentally say the sound MAA. *Continue for up to 11 min.*

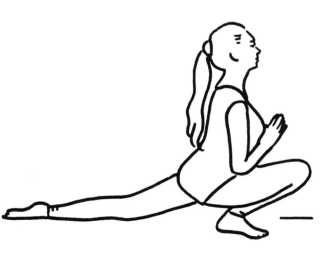

Comments
This is known as **Siam Kriya.** Besides being good for the parathyroid, mastery of this kriya is said to impart the secret of "nothingness and everything."
See also "Thyroid Gland Imbalance."

Phobias—see "Addiction"

Piles—see "Urethritis"

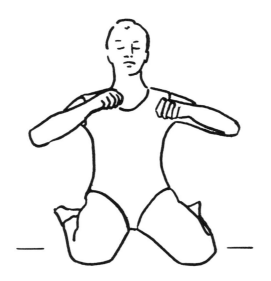

Pimples—see "Colon, to Cleanse"

Pineal Gland Imbalance
(1 1/2 min)

Sit in celibate pose, heels just to the sides of the buttocks. Place your thumbs on the mounds just below the little fingers of each hand and close the fingers over the thumbs in a fist. Place the fists in front of the chest and rotate them very rapidly around each other, making circles away from the body. Concentrate with rapt attention on your rotating hands. Rotate the hands so fast that the motion becomes mechanical. *Continue for 1 1/2 min.*

Comments
This **Drishtee Traatkaa** exercise improves the function of the pineal gland.

Pituitary Gland Imbalance
(1-3 min)

Stand up. As you rapidly alternate from standing on tiptoes to heels-on-floor position, do breath of fire **(a)**. *Continue for 1-3 min.* Then inhale and sit down quickly in easy pose **(b)**, giving a slight jolt to the spine as you do so.

Comments
Don't do this exercise if you have back problems. A set of exercises for the pituitary gland can be found in **Keeping Up with Kundalini Yoga,** pp. 26-27.

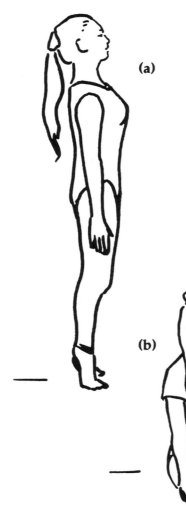

(a)

(b)

Premature Ejaculation
(2-6 min)

1. Lie down on your stomach. Place your palms on the floor beside your shoulders and arch up into cobra pose, **tops** of the feet on the floor. Bring your body up **(1a)** and down **(1b)** as if you were having intercourse. Root lock will automatically be applied. *Continue for 1-3 min.*

2. Sit up with the soles of the feet together in front of you. Put your hands in front of you on the floor, and shift your weight forward till you're balanced on the sides of your feet and your hands. Buttocks are off the floor. Begin bouncing. Feel horny and think of having intercourse. *Continue for 1-3 min.*

Comments
These exercises help men overcome the problem of premature ejaculation. They should be practiced once in the morning and once in the evening. A yogic variation of Exercise 2 is to insert the penis into the area formed by the two joined arches of the feet.

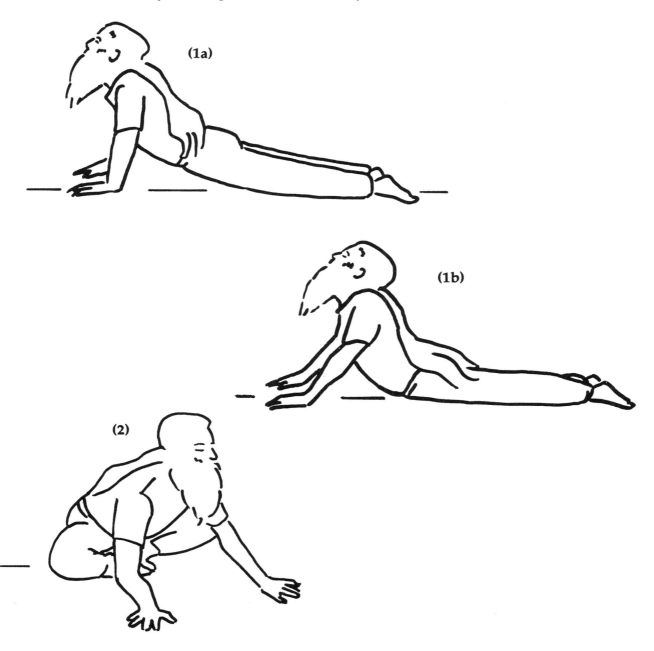

(1a)

(1b)

(2)

Premenstrual Syndrome, for Prevention and Alleviation
(4 min)

In a standing position with knees and heels together, feet flat on the floor and angled out to the sides for balance, raise your arms straight overhead, close to the ears, with palms forward. The thumbs can be locked together. Keeping the legs straight, bend back from the base of the spine 20°. The head, spine, and arms form an unbroken curve, the arms being in line with the ears **(a)**. Hold the posture with long, deep, gentle breath *for 2 min.*

From this position, **very slowly** bend over as far as possible, keeping the arms straight and close to the ears **(b)**. Inhale and, with the breath held in as long as possible, pump the navel point. Then exhale and do the same on the held exhalation. Continue this process *for 2 min.*

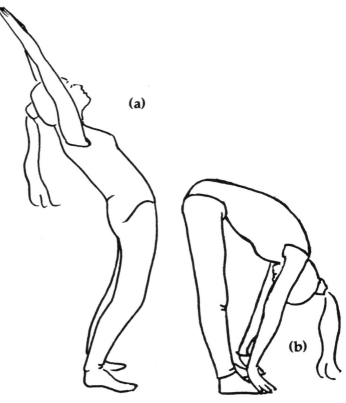

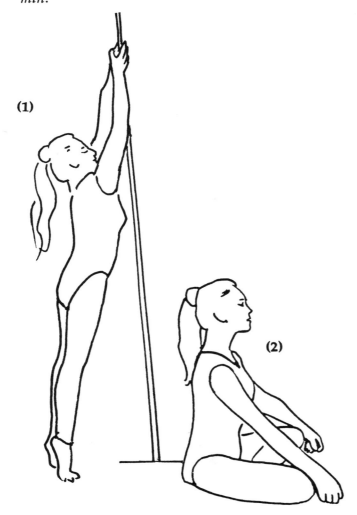

Comments

These 2 exercises help prevent premenstrual syndrome, which is characterized by bodily discomfort, a feeling of insecurity, and emotional behavior just before the onset of the menstrual period. They are also helpful in preventing the onset of **menopause.**

See also "Menstrual Pain." For a set of exercises dealing with premenstrual syndrome, see the **Yoga Manual,** pp. 30-34.

Radiation, to Protect Against
(3 or 11 min)

These are 2 separate exercises:

1. Grab a pole or tree with both arms and stretch yourself. Isometrically tighten your neck muscles—imagine that they are so hard a sword will not cut through them. *Continue for 3 min.*

2. Keeping your teeth together, breathe through a small hole in your mouth. Listen to your breath. *Continue for 3 or 11 min.*

Comments

This meditation strengthens the parathyroid gland, which helps protect us from radiation. The parathyroid will not function properly unless the neck is totally aligned with the spine.

Rashes—see "Colon, to Cleanse"

Sacrum, Stiff—see "Gas, in Men"

Sciatica, to Avoid
(2 min)

Lie down on your back. Bring your body up into shoulder stand, supporting your back with your hands. Keep your body as straight as possible throughout the exercise. Spreading the legs as wide as possible, do breath of fire *for 2 min.* Then inhale completely, and exhale deeply as you relax out of the posture.

Comments
See also "Ovaries, to Relax," and **Sadhana Guidelines,** p. 51, for a set of exercises for the sciatic ("life") nerve.

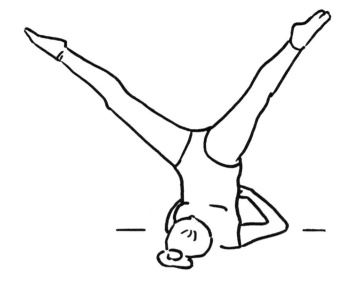

Sexual Frustration—see "Tennis Elbow"

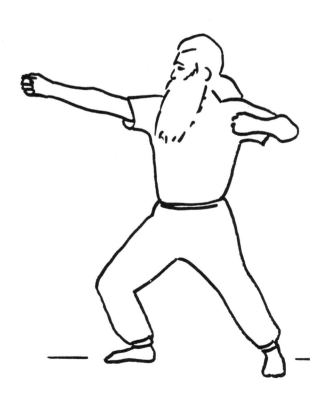

Sexual Glands—see "Heart Attacks, to Prevent"

Sexual Potency
(6-10 min)

Stand with the right leg bent forward enough so that the toes can't be seen over the knee. The left leg is straight back, with the foot flat on the floor at a 45° angle to the front foot. Raise the right arm straight in front, parallel to the floor. Make a fist as if grasping a bow. Pull your left arm back as if pulling a bowstring back to the shoulder. Create a tension across the chest.

Face forward. Fix the eyes above the front fist to the horizon. Hold the position *for 3-5 min*, then switch legs and arms and *repeat*.

Comments
Sat Kriya (Appendix A) is also good for male potency. For more exercises dealing with this topic, see **Relax and Rejoice,** Vol. 2, pp. 24-32. Sets of exercises can be found in the **Yoga Manual** (sexual strength, pp. 18-19) and the **Sadhana Guidelines** (sexual energy, p. 51).

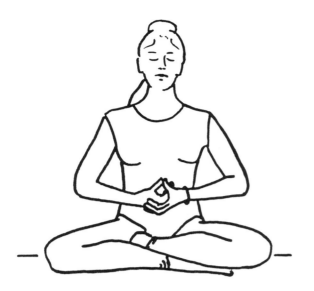

Shock, Sudden
(11-31 min)

Sit straight. Relax the arms down, elbows bent. Draw the forearms in toward each other until the hands meet in front of the body about 1 inch above the navel. Point both palms up and rest the right hand in the palm of the left hand. Pull the thumbs toward the body and press the tips of the thumbs together. Look at the tip of your nose. Deeply inhale. Then completely exhale as you chant the following mantra in a monotone:

**SAT NAAM SAT NAAM SAT NAAM SAT NAAM
SAT NAAM SAT NAAM WAAHE GUROO
SAT NAAM SAT NAAM SAT NAAM SAT NAAM
SAT NAAM SAT NAAM WAAHE GUROO
SAT NAAM SAT NAAM SAT NAAM SAT NAAM
SAT NAAM SAT NAAM WAAHE GUROO**

The entire mantra must be chanted in only one breath! Use the tip of the tongue to pronounce each word exactly. The rhythm must also be exact:

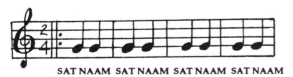

SAT NAAM SAT NAAM SAT NAAM SAT NAAM

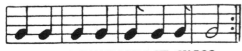

SAT NAAM SAT NAAM WAA-HE GU-ROO

Begin with 11 min, and slowly build up to 31 min with practice. Upon completion of the meditation, deeply inhale and completely exhale 5 times. Then deeply inhale, hold the breath, and stretch the arms up over the head as high as possible. Stretch with every ounce that you can muster. Exhale and relax down. Repeat twice.

Comments

This meditation balances the Western hemisphere of the brain with the base of the Eastern hemisphere. This enables the brain to maintain its equilibrium under **stress** or after a sudden shock. It also keeps the nerves from being shattered under those circumstances.

Shoulders, Stiff
(3 min)

Sit in easy pose. Place the hands on the knees. Rotate the shoulders either forward or backward *for 3 min.* Do your best to get maximum rotation—forward, up, back, and down.

Comments

Shoulder rolls help remove calcium deposits ("crystals") in the shoulders.

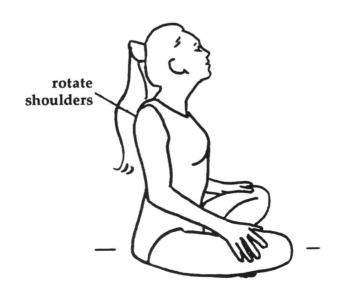

rotate shoulders

Sinuses, to Clear
(2-6 min)

Sit with your feet straight out in front of you. Put your right foot on top of your left thigh. Catch the left toe with both hands (or the ankle if you can't reach the toe). Inhale. Exhale and bring your body down toward your left knee. Inhale up again.

Continue *for 1-3 min*, then switch sides and begin again.

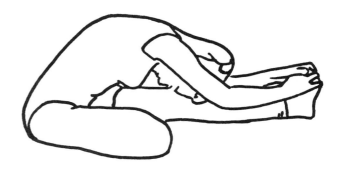

Skin Problems—see "Colon, to Cleanse"; "Thyroid Gland Imbalance"

Smoking—see "Addiction"

Spine, Lower, Problems

See "Adrenal Gland Imbalance." For sets of exercises dealing with the lower spine, see the **Sadhana Guidelines,** pp. 52 and 61-62.

Spine, Stiff—see "Aging"

Spleen, to Strengthen
(5 min)

Lie on your back. Raise your legs to 90° and cross the ankles. In this position, do long, deep breathing as you wiggle your toes. *Continue for 5 min.*

Comments
See also "Gallbladder Problems"; "Heart Attacks, to Prevent."

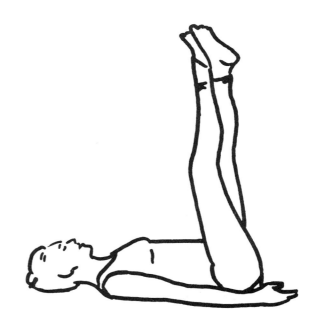

Stomach Pain—see "Digestive Problems, Emergency"

Stress–see "Adrenal Gland Imbalance"; "Shock, Sudden"

Sympathetic Nervous System, to Repair
(11 min maximum)

Sit in easy pose with a straight spine. Touch the tip of the ring finger of each hand to the corresponding thumb **(ravi mudra)**. Extend both arms parallel to the floor with the palms down. Spread the fingers wide. Put the sides of the tips of the index fingers together. Raise the arms slightly so the index fingernails are at the level of the eyes. Keep the eyes relaxedly open. Look over the index fingertips to the horizon **(1)**. Just hold this position completely still. *Continue for up to 11 min,* **but no longer.**

Comments
Otherwise known as the Meditation for Human Quality, this kriya balances and repairs the sympathetic nervous system. It also helps the heart, and gives resistance to **tension** and high pressure environments. Its greatest result is to connect you with the inner sense of being human by enhancing the qualities of endurance, creativity, and compassion.

Tennis Elbow
(3 min)

Come into **frog pose:** Squat down so your buttocks are on your heels, with the heels off the floor and touching each other. Put the fingertips on the floor between the knees. Keep the head up **(2a)**. Inhale as you raise the buttocks high, keeping the fingertips on the floor and the heels together. In the "up" position, the head should be facing the knees **(2b)**. Exhale strongly, coming down and allowing the buttocks to strike the heels. *Continue for 3 min.*

Comments
In ancient India, a man was not considered marriageable if he could not do frog pose for 2 1/2 hours without a rest! Besides **transforming sexual energy** for use in the higher chakras, regular practice of this exercise helps prevent tennis elbow. It is good for the **heart,** the **hearing** and the **eyesight.** It flushes the **arteries** and the **lymph system.** The practice of this kriya also flushes the breasts with blood, helping prevent **breast cancer** in women.

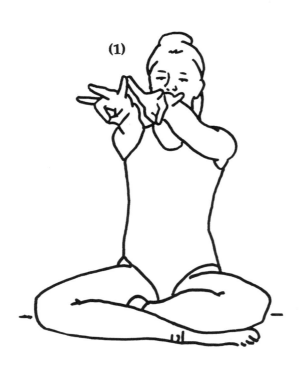

(1)

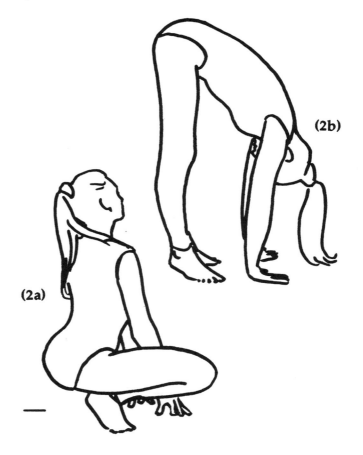

(2a) (2b)

Tension

(about 7 min)

Sit in rock pose, hands on your knees. Lean back to 60° from the horizontal, head relaxed back **(3a)**. Do long, deep breathing *for 2 min*. Then inhale, and hold the breath in as long as possible. (Don't make yourself faint, though.) Exhale and relax.

Put your hands in Venus lock under the hair, against the skin of the back of the neck. Lean forward, spine straight **(3b)**. Hold the position *for 2 min*.

Sit up in regular rock pose **(3c)**. Inhale and exhale 3 times deeply. On the last exhale, hold the breath out as long as possible as you pull root lock and concentrate your eyes and your attention on the crown chakra at the top of the head. *Repeat this exercise 2 more times.*

Sit with your legs spread wide. Catch the big toes with the thumb and forefinger of each hand and hold on tight **(3d)**. With a straight spine, inhale deeply, exhale completely, and pull root lock as you look to your third-eye point. Do this inhale–exhale–lock *a total of 3 times*. Then relax.

Comments

See also "Heart Problems"; "Sympathetic Nervous System, to Repair." Other exercises for and information on tension can be found in **StressAway—The Way to Relax**. The **Survival Kit** contains a meditation to neutralize tension (p. 39).

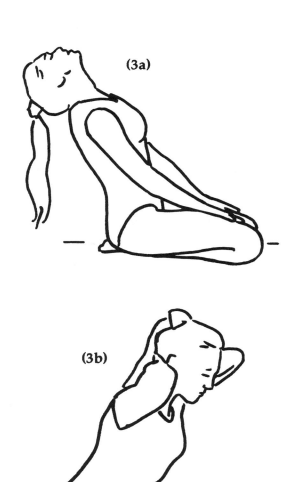

(3a)

(3b)

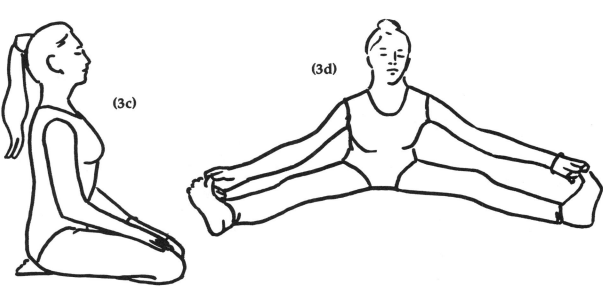

(3c)

(3d)

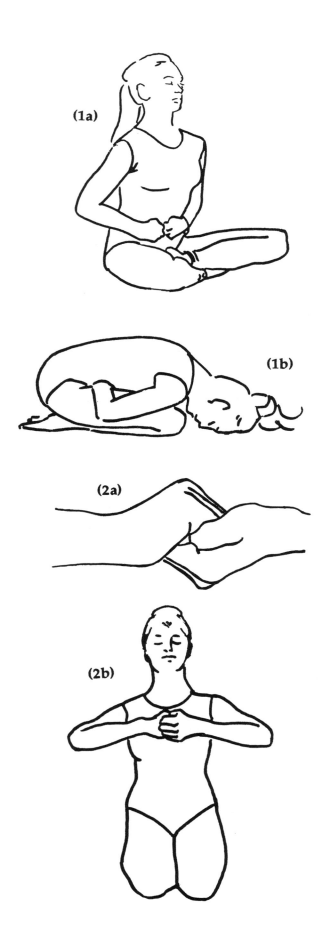

(1a)

(1b)

(2a)

(2b)

Throat, Sore
(34 min)

Sit on your heels, hands in fists, knuckles pressed into the navel **(1a)**. Bring your forehead to the floor **(1b)**. Do breath of fire *for 3 min*, then long, deep breathing *for 31 min*.

Thymus Gland Imbalance
(1-3 min)

Sit on your heels. Place the hands in bear grip **(2a)** at chest level with the forearms parallel to the floor **(2b)**. Inhale. Hold the breath, and without separating the hands, try to pull the hands apart. Apply maximum force. Exhale. Inhale and pull again. *Continue for 1-3 min*. Then inhale, exhale, and relax.

Comments

Besides stimulating the thymus gland, this exercise opens the heart center.

Thyroid Gland Imbalance
(1-3 min)

Stand up, hands in prayer mudra at the chest, elbows relaxed at the sides **(3a)**. Inhale deeply and extend the arms up and back to 60° from the horizontal, dropping your head back **(3b)**. Exhale as you return to the original position. *Continue for 1-3 min*.

Comments

Along with the **parathyroid gland,** the thyroid gland is the guardian of health and beauty. Improper balance of these 2 glands can make you age before your time. The **skin,** the **complexion,** and the outward appearance are affected by the thyroid.

See also "Gas, in Men." A meditation to balance the thyroid gland can be found in the **Yoga Manual,** p. 27. A meditation to stimulate both the thyroid and the parathyroid can be found in the **Meditation Manual,** p. 60 (I).

Tranquilizer

(3 min)

Sit in easy pose with a straight spine. With the elbows bent, bring the hands up and in until they meet in front of the body at the level of the heart. The elbows should be held up almost to the level of the hands. Bend the index fingers of each hand in toward the palm. Join them with each other so they press together along the second joint. The middle fingers are extended and meet at the fingertips. The other fingers are curled into the hand. The thumbs meet at the fingertips **(4a)**. Hold the mudra about 4 inches from the body with the extended fingers pointing away from the body **(4b)**.

Focus on the tip of your nose. Inhale completely and hold the breath in while mentally repeating the mantra of your choice (SAT NAAM or WAAHE GUROO would be fine) 11-21 times. Then exhale, hold the breath out, and repeat the mantra an equal number of times. *Continue this practice for 3 min.*

Comments

This meditation can tranquilize the mind in 3 min. The hand position is called "the mudra that pleases the mind." Buddha is said to have given it to his disciples for control of the mind.

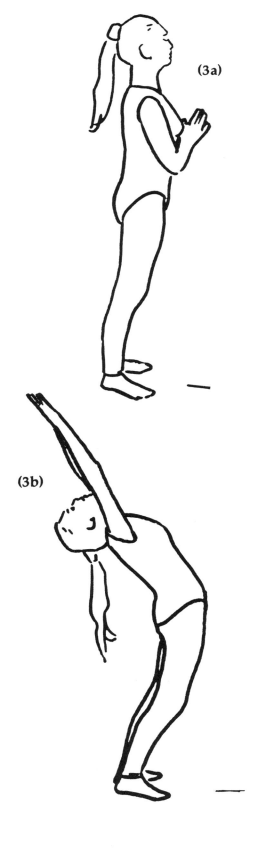

(3a)

(3b)

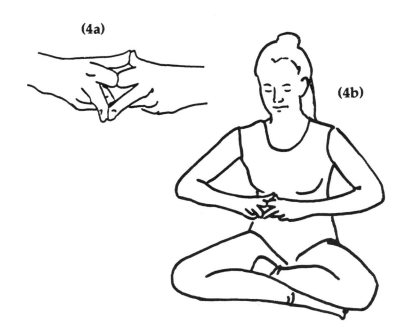

(4a)

(4b)

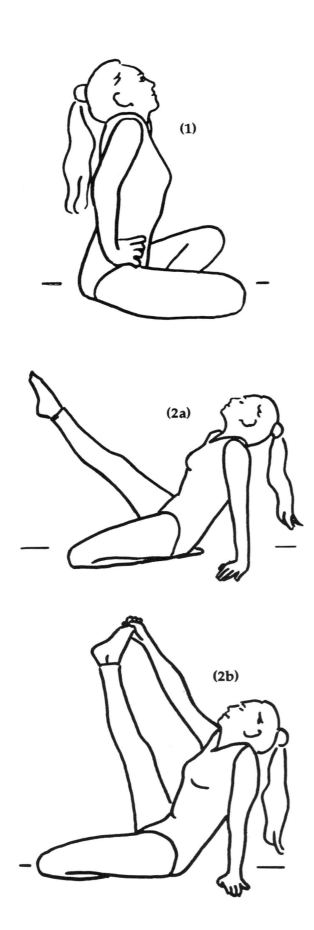

Tuberculosis
(1-3 min)

Sit in easy pose, hands on the hips. Pull the navel in and raise the shoulders as high as you can **(1)**. *Continue for 1-3 min.*

Urethritis
(about 4-8 min)

Sit with your left heel at the rectum, right leg extended out in front. Placing palms on the floor behind you, lean back and bring your right leg up as high as possible **(2a).** Inhale completely. Exhale completely, hold the air out, and pull root lock. Inhale and relax.

Still sitting on the left heel, grab the right ankle or heel with the right hand. Leaning back on your left palm **(2b),** inhale completely. Exhale completely, and pull root lock on the held exhalation. Inhale and relax.

Come into **frog pose:** Squat down so the buttocks rest on the heels. Heels are off the floor and touching each other throughout the exercise. Put the fingertips on the floor between the knees. Head is up, gazing forward **(2c).** Now inhale as you raise the buttocks high, keeping the fingers on the floor. At the height of the inhalation you should be looking at your knees **(2d).** Exhale as you come back down into the crouching position. Do this cycle *a total of 30 times.* Then inhale up, hold the breath in briefly, exhale, and relax.

Comments
This set is excellent for urethritis and for **hemorrhoids (piles).**

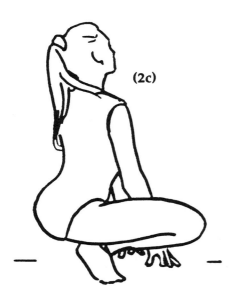

(2c)

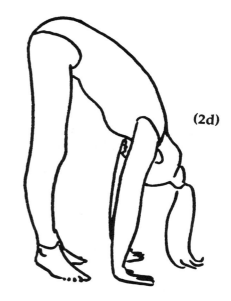

(2d)

Varicose Veins
(2 min)

Stand up straight. Put the hands on the back of the thighs and lean back **(3a).** Sit down in easy pose **(3b),** then immediately stand up and lean back again.

Continue as rapidly as possible *for 2 min.*

Weakness—see "Fever"

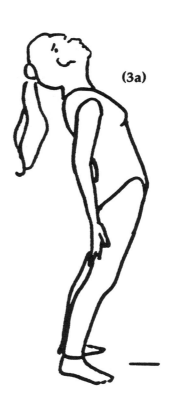

(3a)

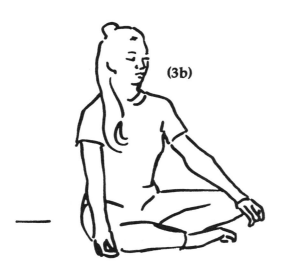

(3b)

Wet Dreams, to Prevent
(3-5 min)

This exercise requires a fair amount of flexibility. Sit between the heels in celibate pose. Carefully lower yourself back onto the floor. Extend the hands straight up over the head, perpendicular to the floor, palms flat together. Begin Sat Kriya in this position. Repeat the mantra SAT NAAM at a slow, steady pace. When you say SAT, pull up and in slightly on the navel point and pull root lock. When you say NAAM, relax the navel and the lock. Visualize energy flowing from the base of the spine through the top of the skull with each repetition of the mantra.

Continue for 3-5 min. When you finish the exercise, relax out of the posture slowly, taking care not to jerk your muscles.

Note: The posture indicated for Sat Kriya in the above exercise is unusual. See Appendix A for the standard version of Sat Kriya, including comments relevant to both versions.

Youthfulness, to Regain
(3, 11, or 31 min)

Sitting in easy pose, with spine straight and chin pressed slightly back toward the back of the neck, place hands on knees, index finger and tip of thumb of each hand touching. Roll the tongue back towards its root and suck on it (**manduki mudra**). In a short time, a nectar-like flow will begin in the mouth. Patiently drink it.

Continue for 3, 11, or 31 min.

Comments
If practiced regularly, this kriya achieves **youthfulness** of the flesh, **regenerates muscle**, and makes **grey hair** disappear. Raise the length of time you practice it to the point where you feel fulfilled *(up to 31 min maximum)*. Good effects of this kriya are subject to the condition that you have a moderate sex life and a good diet.

See also "Aging"; "Blood Disease." For a youthfulness set, see the **Sadhana Guidelines**, pp. 55-56.

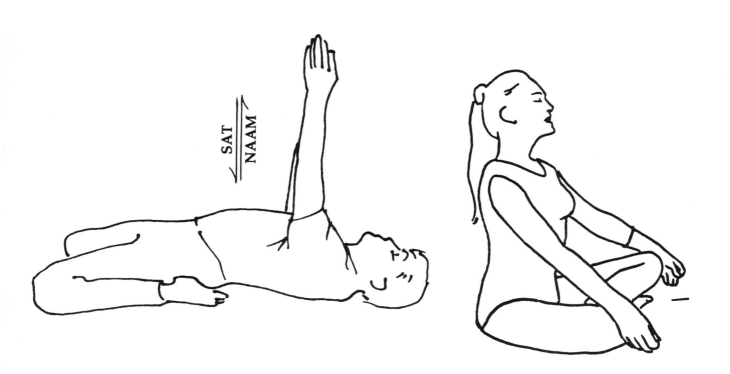

SAT / NAAM

5. HEALING OTHERS

Those who send good vibrations out will receive them 10 times over from the universe. You gain when you give. There is no need to pray for yourself—pray for others and the Creator will pray for you.

—Yogi Bhajan

There are situations, as in the case of a young child or a friend either too ill or too set in his or her ways, when the person who is ill cannot do yoga to speed the healing process. In such situations, it is possible for you, as a concerned friend or relative, to practice various techniques through which healing energy (prana) can be accumulated and transferred to the one who is sick. Such techniques, which are the subject of this chapter, have the added advantage of improving the health of the sender, as one must first be healthy in order to impart health. Most of the meditations in this chapter can be done by just one person. One is to be done by a group, and one is a meditation against burnout, the depletion of body energy that sometimes results when one's natural healing ability is overworked.

For simple, healing massage techniques, see **Healing through Yoga, Meditation, and Massage,** pp. 5-6 and 11-13. See Appendix C for details.

BEGINNERS' MEDITATIONS TO BECOME SENSITIVE TO AND TRANSFER PRANIC ENERGY

Becoming Sensitive to Prana
(5 min or so)

Sit in easy pose. Raise your hands and massage the fingers into the palms until you feel a tingling sensation **(a).** Next, place the palms, facing each other and about 6 inches apart, in front of the chest. Keep the fingers straight and the hands stiff **(b).** Concentrate on the energy passing from one hand to the other, and visualize the spinal column as a beautiful, shining cord of energy. *Continue for 3-4 min.*

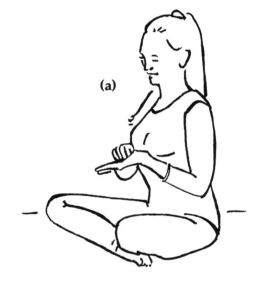

(a)

Extend the arms out straight to the sides, palms outward **(c).** Feel the center of the palms being charged with energy, then concentrate on any part of your body that is sick and direct the incoming energy there. *Continue for 1-3 min.* Then relax.

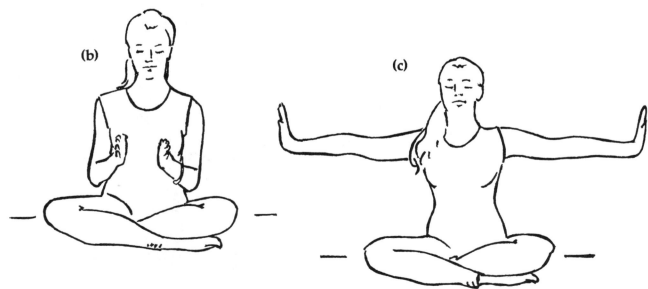

(b)

(c)

Transferring Energy
(15-18 min)

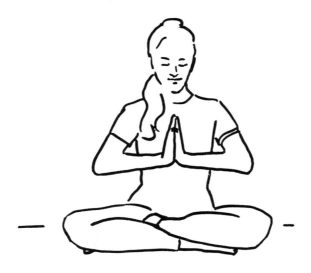

Sitting in easy pose, place the hands together at the center of the chest (prayer mudra). Press the hands together with all the power you can muster, and concentrate on the heart chakra. Let hate depart; fill the heart with love. *Continue for 4-5 min.*

Now think of someone you love very much and send them healing thoughts. Healing thoughts can be transmitted like radio waves; fill the whole room with them. Project them to the person you love.

Concentrate in this way *for at least 10 min.* Then inhale deeply, fill your chest with love, and project pranic energy like a thunderbolt to the one you love. Exhale, inhale, and send the energy of this breath to the person on whom you are meditating. Exhale. Inhale again, and feel energy flowing from your hands to the person. Create a mental link. Feel the energy massaging the person. Exhale. Inhale and continue *for 1-3 min.* Then exhale and relax.

DHRIB DHRISTI LOCHINA KARMA MEDITATION
FOR HEALING EYES
(15 min to 2 1/2 hours; best practiced on the eve of the full moon)

Sit in easy pose with a straight spine, hands in gyan mudra on the knees. The shoulders and hips should be in line. Now lock the tips of the front teeth together. Focus the eyes on the tip of the nose. The tongue touches the upper palate (this should occur automatically within about a minute). Project the mantra SAA TAA NAA MAA (*aa* as in "far") out from the third-eye point. Beam it out, creating an internal harmony.

Continue for 31 min. Minimum compromise time is 15 min; if you wish to master it, practice for 1 1/2 hours at a sitting. Three hours' practice at a sitting are said to open up psychic abilities.

Comments
The name of this very powerful, but simple, meditation means "the action of acquiring insight into the future." Honest practice of this kriya is said to impart many benefits in addition to the power to heal with the eyes. According to tradition, your words will have the power to penetrate deeply; you will learn to talk inspiringly and your words will always represent the truth of a given situation; you will be able to project your personality or your bodily sensations anywhere; and you will always know the consequence of any sequence of actions that you start.

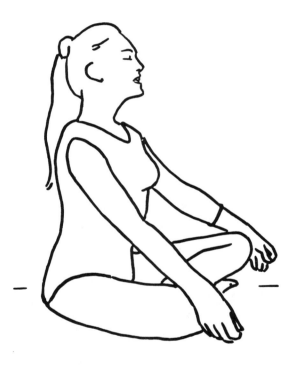

When practiced on the eve of the full moon, the kriya is said to influence the subconscious mind most completely. While most meditations require long periods of practice for mastery, it is possible to master this kriya in one or several sittings. Concentrate with total devotion!

106

HALF STAR-OF-DAVID MEDITATION
TO BECOME A NATURAL HEALER
(11 min, building to 31 min with practice)

Sit in rock pose, in easy pose, or on a chair with the weight equally distributed on both feet. Place the hands at heart level, arms relaxed near the sides of the body. The thumb and first two fingers of each hand are pressed against the corresponding thumb and fingers of the other hand with a pressure firm enough to produce great heat in the hands. The thumbs are pressed straight back towards the heart. The first two fingers point up and away from the chest at an angle of about 60° from the floor. The other two fingers are not touching; separate them down and apart from each other.

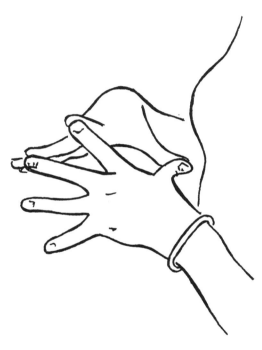

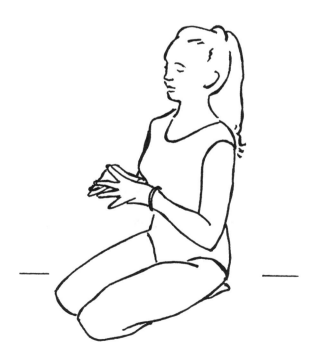

With eyelids closed, look up toward the top of the skull. Breathe very slowly, very deeply, and very consciously through the nose. Attach your favorite mantra (for example, SAT NAAM or WAAHE GUROO) to the breath. Imagine a healing light flowing with your breath.

Continue for 11 min maximum at the first sitting. You may add 1 min for every 2 or 3 days of practice up to a total of 31 min.

Comments

It is said that this meditation was given by Sarah to Hazarath Abraham, guardian of the Jews, when he went to Egypt. It is considered to make its practitioner perfectly healthy and wise, and a very beautiful natural healer.

MEDITATION FOR HEALING POWER
IN THE HANDS
(3, 11, or 31 min)

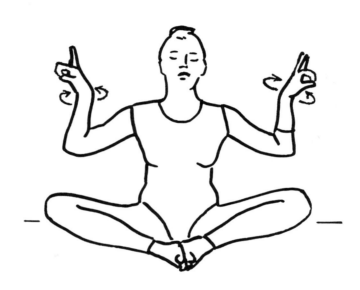

Sit either in easy pose or in **butterfly pose** (soles of the feet touching and drawn in toward the groin). Hands are in gyan mudra with the upper arms extending out from the sides of the body and parallel to the ground. Forearms point straight up throughout the meditation. The hands **(only)** rotate in a snappy action in and out in rhythm with the following mantra, which is chanted over and over in a monotone:

Mantra: WAAHE GUROO WAAHE GUROO
Hands: in   out   in   out

Mantra: WAAHE WAAHE WAAHE GUROO
Hands: in   out   in   out

Continue for 3, 11, or 31 min.

Comments

This meditation is reputed to give healing power in the hands. As you practice it you may experience a feeling of heat in the hands, then in the arms, the back of the neck, and finally the top of the head.

Other good meditations for healing power in the hands can be found in the **Meditation Manual**, p. 60 (II), and in **Healing through Yoga, Meditation, and Massage**, pp. 7-10. See Appendix C for details.

DOI ASHTAPADI JAP MEDITATION
TO HEAL THROUGH THE SPIRIT
(11-31 min)

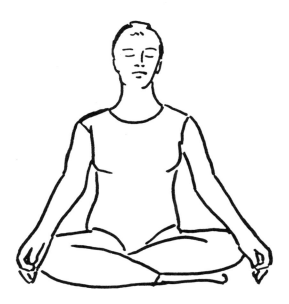

Sit straight in either easy pose or lotus pose. Put the hands in gyan mudra and rest them on the knees. Concentrating on the third-eye point, begin long, deep breathing. On the inhalation, mentally vibrate the mantra SAT NAAM 16 times. On the exhalation, vibrate the mantra WAAHE GUROO 16 times. Do the mental chant in groups of 4: 4 strokes up, then 4 down. this will help you keep the count and the rhythm in your mind. The rhythm should be constant, like water dripping quickly off the eaves of a house.

Begin with 11 min of meditation and increase about 2 min a day until you reach 31 min.

Comments

This very famous kriya is said to have been taught by Jesus of Nazareth as a method of attaining Christ consciousness. For that reason, and also because it is done in 32 parts, a number identified in numerology with Christ, it is also known as the **Christ mantra.**

Indian scriptures state that all sickness leaves and all bad omens fall away from a person when this meditation is practiced. The chant balances the forces of prana and apana and energizes the sushumna. That allows one's life to be longer and well balanced. Honest mastery of this meditation is also said to confer the power to heal through the hands. Do the meditation with love and devotion.

RAA MAA DAA SAA MEDITATION
TO HEAL SELF OR OTHERS
(11 min beginning; up to 31 min with practice)

Sit in easy pose, elbows in snug at your sides, forearms snug against your upper arms, fingers together and pulled down and out so that the palms are parallel with and facing the ceiling. Close your eyes nine-tenths.

Inhale completely, then exhale completely as you chant the following mantra:

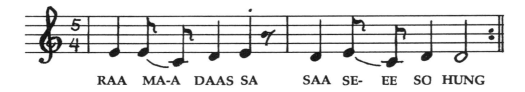

RAA   MA-A   DAAS SA   SAA   SE-   EE   SO   HUNG

As you chant SA, the navel point is pulled in, so that this syllable is abbreviated. The other syllables are drawn out in a strong, powerful chant that uses all the breath with each repetition of the mantra. Strive to maintain your chant at full volume (loud, but not raucous) throughout the meditation.

Continue for 11 min. Very gradually, over a period of **years,** the time may be increased to a maximum of 31 min.

Comments

This highly effective meditation deals with **Vayu Siddhi,** the power of air. It brings health and many other desirable positive changes. If you wish to heal yourself, imagine a glowing green light around yourself as you meditate. If you wish to heal someone else, imagine that same light around the other person as you meditate.

A variation of this chant with a different mudra can be found in the **Survival Kit,** p. 29. See Appendix C for details.

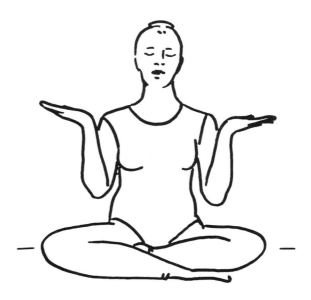

MEDITATION AGAINST BURNOUT
(11, 22, or 31 min)

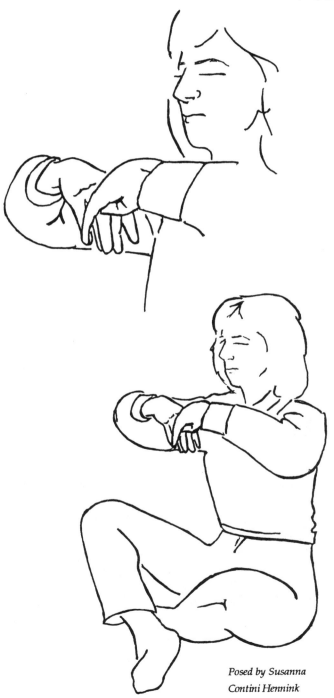

Posed by Susanna
Contini Hennink

This meditation should be practiced only when there is time after completion to remain still and relaxed, as it can leave you feeling very spaced out. Sit in easy pose with a straight spine. Relax the arms down with the elbows bent. Raise the forearms up and in toward each other until the backs of the hands meet at the level of the heart, fingers pointing toward the floor. Fold the thumbs across the palms until the tip of the thumb of each hand rests at the base of the ring finger. Firmly press the backs of the hands together in the area of the knuckles. (The upper hands may be more loosely pressed together.) Keep the arms comfortable and relaxed, and the elbows as loose as possible.

Focus on the tip of your nose. Deeply inhale in 8 equal parts. Completely exhale in 8 equal parts. There is no mantra for this meditation. However, during group practice the leader can call out SAA TAA NAA MAA, SAA TAA NAA MAA . . . to establish the rhythm and power of the 8-stroke inhalation and exhalation.

Begin with 11 min of practice. When you feel competent, increase to 22 min. Later, increase to 31 min.

Comments

The mudra of this meditation brings about a dormant state of energy so that you can either prevent burnout or recuperate. The posture keeps your magnetic field concentrated within itself. For a set of exercises to prevent burnout, see the **Sadhana Guidelines,** p. 74. See Appendix C for details.

HEALING RING OF THE TANTRA
(11 or 31 min)

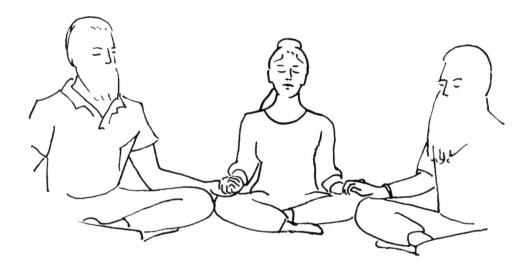

This meditation is only to be done on the following days: full moon, new moon, or eleventh day of the new moon. It should not be practiced with less than 11 people. Moreover, during the meditation the ring must never be broken for any reason.

A group of 11 or more persons sits round in a circle in any comfortable, cross-legged position, spines straight. All participants hold hands with the persons sitting next to them, forming an unbroken circle. The eyes are closed.

One person begins by sweetly and powerfully calling the words WAAHE GUROO in a monotone. WAA and HE each have one beat, and GUROO has two beats. Once this mantra has been called out, the other members of the circle answer with WAAHE GUROO, chanting as described above. The caller then says SAT NAAM softly, and the person sitting to the left of the caller becomes the next caller, who then calls out WAAHE GUROO. The others answer WAAHE GUROO, the caller says SAT NAAM softly, and the next person to the left becomes caller, with the chant continuing in a clockwise direction around the circle.

Inhale as the mantra is being chanted by the caller; exhale as you chant the mantra in response (unless, of course, you're the caller). *Continue for at least 11 min*, and preferably 31 min.

Comments

This healing ring can be used to generate and direct tremendous healing energy towards any person—a member of the circle, someone at a far distance, or someone located in the center of the circle. The participants should focus their minds on listening, and let themselves be filled with the sound, acutely tuning in to the call, and then answering.

Appendix A. Healing Lifestyles

Diet

Sun, Earth, and Ground Foods

In India, foods are divided into **sun foods, earth foods,** and **ground foods.** Sun foods grow more than three feet from the ground. Fruits, nuts, avocados, dates, and coconuts are sun foods. They make the body and nervous system quick and light. They are good for people with big bones and for slow-moving people. Old people need more of them and less heavy foods and grains.

Earth foods grow under the soil. Radishes, beets, carrots, potatoes, turnips, onions, garlic, ginger, and peanuts are some of the earth foods. They are good for people with small bones and tall, thin bodies, and for people with nervous dispositions. It is generally good to eat more earth foods in the winter, or when the weather is cold.

Then there are vegetables and those fruits that grow just above the ground. They are part sun, part earth. Most "ground foods" are cleansing foods, and are good steamed, stewed, or fresh.

Raw and Cooked Foods

Raw foods—salads, fruits and some vegetables that are good raw—give us vitamins and minerals and roughage for good elimination. But it is important to eat cooked foods as well. From cooked foods we get some metals and minerals that our body can't obtain from food that is raw. Also, too much raw food can clog the ileocecal valve, a small valve between the small and large intestines. In India they have a special way of cooking using predigested foods and spices and oils to give the body warmth and energy. Ripe fruits and raw vegetables are also used for balance. This way of cooking is very good for digestion and elimination.[1]

> ## Water for Health
>
> Drinking 8 glasses of water a day will flush your body of toxins and help it stay healthy. Be sure to drink water before bedtime, as dehydration during sleep can cause irritation and bad dreams.

Acidity and Alkalinity

People in India believe that when the blood is slightly alkaline a person will be calm and happy. When the blood is acidic the body can get ill or age quickly. Whether the blood is alkaline or acid depends on diet. Sweet and sour fruit, green vegetables, pulses and legumes (peas, beans, lentils, and so on), milk, yogurt, curd, and buttermilk make the blood alkaline. Although citric fruits like lemons are acidic, they make the blood alkaline. These foods keep the organs, nerves, and glands healthy. They keep us healthy, calm, able to overcome our troubles without just reacting to them.

----
[1]See **Golden Temple Vegetarian Cookbook** and **From Vegetables, with Love,** two excellent Indian cookbooks for health maintenance (Appendix C).

Pre-Digested Food

This recipe for mung beans and rice is high in protein, inexpensive, and easy on the digestive system.

1 cup mung beans (health food store)
1 cup Basmati rice (health food store or Indian grocery)
9 cups water
4-6 cups chopped assorted vegetables (carrots, celery, zucchini, broccoli, etc.)
2 onions, chopped
1/3 cup minced ginger root
8-10 cloves garlic, minced
1 heaping teaspoon turmeric
1/2 teaspoon pepper
1 heaping teaspoon garam masala (health food store or Indian grocery)
1 teaspoon crushed red chilies
1 tablespoon sweet basil
2 bay leaves
seeds of 5 cardamom pods
salt or soy sauce to taste
(yogurt or cheese)

Rinse beans and rice. Bring water to a boil, add rice and beans, and let boil over a medium flame. Prepare vegetables and add them to the cooking rice and beans. Heat about 1/2 cup oil in a large frying pan. Add onions, garlic, and ginger and saute over a medium-high flame until they begin to brown. Add spices, but not salt and herbs. When nicely done, combine onions with cooking mung beans and rice. Stir often to prevent scorching. Add herbs. Continue to cook, stirring frequently, over a medium-low flame until the consistency is rich, thick, and soup-like, with ingredients barely discernible.

Serve with yogurt, or with cheese melted over the top. *Serves 4-6.*

—Foods for Health and Healing

Meat, fish, eggs, and starches make the blood acid. They give a quick energy lift, but then let us down. Fats like ghee, butter, margarine, and oil are neutral. But because they are hard to digest, they tax the pancreas, gall bladder, and liver.

Our bodies need both alkaline and acid foods. It's a good rule, if you eat meat, to make fish, meat, eggs, and starches only a third of your diet. Vegetarians might want to make rice, bread, sweets, and butter products only a third of their diet. Whether you eat meat or not, it is best to make most of the diet steamed vegetables, fruits, pulses and legumes, nuts, milk, yogurt, and curds. If there is a specific problem, vitamins and protein drinks can be used to supplement a good diet. There are also special foods to correct special problems, such as daikon radish for jaundice.[2]

Spiritual Practice

The stars glitter in the dewy night. The saintly persons, beloved of my Lord, remain awake. The lovers of the omnipresent Lord ever remain wakeful, and night and day remember His name.

—Siri Guru Granth Sahib

Yogic scriptures specify that 2 1/2 hours of spiritual discipline, or **sadhana,** be done before sunrise every day. In the hours just before dawn, life force or prana concentrates in the lungs, brain, and nervous system. Mental balance and physical cleansing are accomplished more easily in these hours than during the rest of the day. The yogis say that only angels are awake at this time, and that the auric protection and guidance of our divine inner light is strongest then. If instead of sleeping we do a spiritual practice, the dreams that crowd the subconscious of the sleeping mind during that time surface through the conscious mind and are released. The less subconscious "garbage" we have, the less pain we will have in our lives. The mind leads the body, and a healthy mind, uncluttered with negativity, creates a healthy body. Sadhana is a "tune-up" for your earthly vehicle. Through it you can tune your mental, physical, and spiritual rhythms to each other.

----

[2]A comprehensive work containing remedies for health is **Foods for Health and Healing,** based on the teachings of Yogi Bhajan. Also available is an advanced text called **The Ancient Art of Self-Healing** (see Appendix C).

Then no part of yourself will be out of step with any other part.

There are many kinds of sadhana, but there is a practical structure of sadhana that gives optimum results. Set aside one area of your living space that can be used only or mainly for sadhana. Keep it clean and neat; place in it objects or pictures that remind you of your higher consciousness. Air should be allowed to circulate and the temperature should be kept moderate. The spot you sit on should be covered with sheepskin or a wool blanket, as these are nonstatic and insulate our magnetic field from that of the earth. If neither of these is available, the next best substance to sit on is wood.

Always fold your hands, palms together, at the center of your chest and chant the words ONG NAMO, GUROO DEV NAMO 3 times before you begin. (See the section on "Tuning In" in Chapter 2.) These words will help you channel the energy you create toward your higher consciousness.

The first half of your sadhana can be spent doing a yoga set. The second half can be spent doing one or several chanting meditations. Some excellent models for sadhana can be found in the **Sadhana Guidelines** (see Appendix C).

When you chant during sadhana, you will feel negative thoughts surfacing from your subconscious mind. It is important not to repress these negative thoughts. If you do, the chant will seal the negative thoughts in your subconscious mind. Instead, let the thoughts come, look at them with your neutral or meditative mind, then just let the thoughts go. Let the chant carry them away. This is the actual mechanism of cleansing the subconscious mind. Meditation can be your daily "psychiatrist" if it is done in this way.

The essence of a good sadhana is constant practice. If you can do it for 40 consecutive days, it will become a habit that can be continued with much less effort than it takes at first.

It is much easier to keep up if you can find family or friends who would like to do it with you. Otherwise, if you would like to try sadhana with a group, contact your local kundalini yoga teaching center (see Appendix B) and ask if you can attend one of their morning sadhanas.

On Coping with Stress

To tell another to relax but not to tell him how
Is to ask a man to till a field then not supply the plow.

—*Anonymous*

We are presently in what historians will probably call the "Age of Stress." That is because changes both in the individual and in society are coming so fast that there is no time to absorb and adjust to them. With the great acceleration of life's pace today, most people's nervous systems have become overloaded. For many people, anxiety is a way of life.

Stress affects everything we do. It affects how well we sleep at night. It affects how alert and energetic we are during the day. It affects what we choose to eat and how we digest it. Our health is linked to our stress level, as stress is the root of such diseases as cancer and heart failure. Our anxiety level also affects our relations with other people. It is impossible to love, be patient, and help other people when our nerves are chronically on edge and our bodies tense. Too much stress also leads to such self-destructive habits as smoking, overeating, drug use, and overworking.

Three things directly affect our stress level. These are diet, exercise, and the ability to maintain a meditative mind. If you are under stress, include in your diet vitamins C, A, D, and E and the B complex, all important in fighting stress. Also take extra calcium and phosphorus, magnesium, iron, and copper. Anti-stress foods include bananas, almonds, raisins, broccoli, spinach, wheat germ, sunflower seeds, and milk and honey. Whenever you feel particularly stressed out, drink a glass of water. It will lower your body temperature subtly, slow your breathing, and make you feel centered.

Foods that a person under stress should avoid are caffeine, which is actually a poison (found in coffee, chocolate, colas, and many teas), white sugar, salt, and nicotine.

For exercises to help deal with stress, see Chapter 4. Doing 11 min of long, deep breathing (Chapter 2) through the left nostril only is also most relaxing. For more on this topic, read Khalsa and Briggs's excellent book **Stress-Away—The Way to Relax** (Appendix C).

Yogi Tea

Yogi tea is a delicious, healthful substitute for coffee or strong, black tea. It can give you a nice high while your feet stay firmly planted on the ground. When regularly included in the diet, it helps correct damage done to the nervous system by drugs and diseases of the nerves. It will improve your memory and balance you out when you're feeling out of balance. It can take away tiredness, discouragement, and depression. Yogi tea is both a remedy and a preventive measure for colds, flu, and diseases of the mucous membranes.

Make at least 4 cups at a time—one is never enough! For each cup use:

10 ounces water
3 cloves (for the nervous system)
seeds of 4 green cardamom pods (for the colon)
4 whole black peppers (a blood purifier)
1/2 stick cinnamon (for the bones)
1 slice ginger root (for the nervous system, colds, flu, and physical weakness)
1/4 teaspoon black tea (to catalyze the other ingredients)
1/2 cup milk (to prevent irritation to the colon and stomach)

Boil the spices for 10-15 min. Add the black tea and steep for 2 min. Add milk, then reheat to the boiling point, remove immediately from the stove, and strain. Add honey to taste.

—Foods for Health and Healing

Anti-Stress Diet Additions

Add to your breakfast:
2 tablespoons wheat germ (over cereal, fruit, or yogurt)
blanched almonds

For mid-morning and mid-afternoon snacks:
1-2 bananas or
1/2 handful each of raisins and sunflower seeds, mixed together

For lunch or dinner add 1 big serving of one of these, at least once a day:
broccoli, steamed
spinach, fresh (in salad) or steamed

Before bed:
1 large glass warm milk and honey

—StressAway—The Way to Relax

Hair

For the hair cells to function optimally, the hair should not be cut or shaved. If you're a woman, putting your hair up in a bun at the top of your head, just over the posterior fontanel, will keep you centered during the day. If you're a man and have long hair, place it in a knot just over the anterior fontanel (midway between the crown of the head and the hairline at the forehead) during the day. If your hair is short, use a head covering of cotton when you are in the sun. (Cotton protects the body's magnetic field.) This will increase secretion by the pineal gland, which functions better when it is screened from sunlight. It will protect the body's electric force as well. And pranic energy will be drawn into the spine, causing the kundalini to rise in balance. As a matter of fact, the word "kundalini" is sometimes translated as "a coil of the beloved's hair"!

Keeping the hair up also protects it. You will find that the ends do not split and become damaged. However, as the hair grows longer, be careful not to directly shampoo the ends of the hair. Wash the scalp area thoroughly; then when you rinse the soap off enough shampoo will be carried to the ends of the hair to keep them clean. Natural oils from the scalp cannot travel all the way down to the ends of very long hair. Therefore, the night before shampooing, rub in almond oil, especially at the ends, and leave it on overnight.

For the same reason, and to protect the body's magnetic field, brush the hair with a natural bristle brush or wooden comb twice a day for 5 min. Start by bending over so that the hair hangs down over the face. Brush or comb forward from the scalp out to the ends of the hair. Then toss the hair back, and sitting upright, brush back from the scalp to the ends of the hair. Never brush the hair while it is wet, as it stretches and breaks more easily then. It's best to let the hair dry naturally, then brush. If you use a hair drier, as haste sometimes demands, be aware that it wreaks havoc on your magnetic field.

Beard

It's most unfortunate that our society considers wearing a beard, in many instances, socially unacceptable. In shaving his beard, a man loses more than his manly appearance. By covering the pranic nerve in the chin, the beard makes a man much less susceptible to what the yogis call "moon energy." Strange as it may seem, a bearded man is frequently less emotional than his shaven counterpart. If you're a man, try the experiment yourself sometime— take note of your mental state while clean-shaven, then let the beard grow, and see how different you feel.

Sleep

As sleep is the action through which the body and mind regenerate themselves, a well thought out, scientific approach to this activity will directly influence your health. Many people

feel that they need 8 hours of sleep a night in order to face the day, but for a number of reasons 4 to 6 hours are actually optimum for most people.

For one thing, less sleep cuts down on the time spent dreaming, which wastes body energy. Especially in the early morning hours, from 4 to 6 a.m., dreams occur which weigh down the subconscious mind and drain our energy. (That is why many spiritual people do their spiritual practice, or sadhana, during these hours. Old people often tune in to this energy change, wake up quite early, and maintain a high energy level as a result throughout the day.) When you oversleep your breath becomes erratic, which can be bad for the health. When you fall into deep sleep immediately, without lengthy preliminary states of semi-dream and dream sleep, maximum rejuvenation takes place.

Deep sleep is the only stage where the physical body, and especially the brain, is revitalized. It lasts for approximately 2 hours of the time spent sleeping. If you can tune in to this stage directly, it is all the sleep you need. To do this, it is necessary to go through special procedures before going to sleep.

Before Bed

Brush the teeth. Clean the mucus from the throat by putting your finger or a toothbrush at the back of your tongue till you gag a little and your eyes begin to water. Spit out the mucus. (If this mucus is not coughed up, the toxins in it will end up in the colon.) Clean the nostrils and place a little almond oil in each of them. Urinate. Drink a glass of water. Wash the feet with cold water, rub them with a coarse towel, and massage them with almond oil. While massaging the feet, detach yourself from the world and tune in to the one creative cosmic power. This will prepare you for deep sleep.

Now lie down on your back and start breathing long and deep, consciously relaxing each part of the body. With every breath, feel the inflow of cosmic energy which lulls you to the wonderful bliss of sleep. Clear the mind of any disturbance. As you feel yourself sinking into sleep, turn onto your right side and let yourself relax into the breath. This will automatically readjust your breath so that you will breathe through the left nostril, which has a calming and cooling effect on the body and brain. It also takes pressure off the heart and lets the stomach and small intestine drain as you sleep.

Bedding

When you sleep with your body pointing north–south, your body is in line with the earth's magnetic field. This creates a subtle drain on your energy and gives rise to troubled dreams. Simply changing your bed so that it faces east–west can greatly improve your sleep. Try it!

The type of bed you sleep on is also important. Soft beds don't build strong people, as the body becomes restless and spends energy tossing and turning. Back problems also result. For restful, satisfying sleep, a firm bed is best. Waterbeds and traditional box-spring and mattress sets are the worst. The best kind of bed for most people is actually a wool carpet, such as an oriental rug, with a sheepskin on it, covered by a clean, white, cotton sheet. If this is too ascetic for you, add foam rubber an inch thick.

When you are prone for long periods of time, the head should be raised slightly using a pillow. This creates enough pressure to keep the blood circulating properly to the feet and legs. For naps of 15-20 min, elevating the feet on pillows complements the flow of blood to the brain and lightly stimulates the pituitary and pineal glands, giving you a brightly refreshed, rejuvenated feeling.

Waking Up

Three types of energy through which the body operates, and only beginning to be recognized by modern science, are the magnetic force, the electric force, and the life force or prana (Chapter 1). All three must be adjusted before getting up from sleep. It is very important to get up before sunrise. Failure to do so disrupts the balance of prana in the body.

When you awaken, and before you even leave your bed, do these 7 exercises:

1. Turn over onto your back. Stretch your hands up over your head **(a)**. This will channel the magnetic energy. Then keep your eyes closed and put your palms over them **(b)**. Open the eyes and slowly raise the hands, focusing your eyes on the palms as you do so **(c)**.

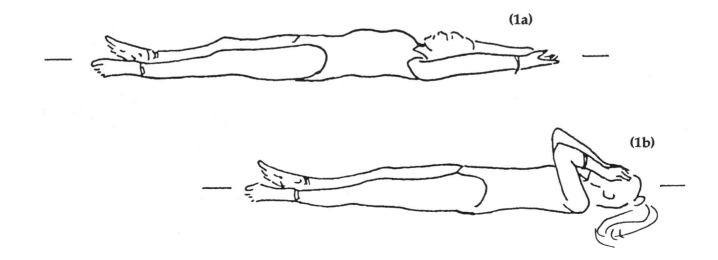

(1a)

(1b)

118

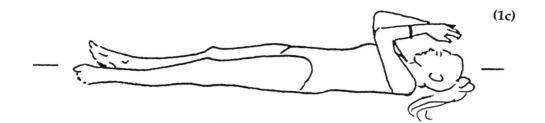

(1c)

2. Begin massaging your face, rubbing from the forehead out to the sides of the eyebrows. Massage the cheeks down to the chin. (Men should continue stroking to the end of the beard.)

3. Do **cat stretch:** While still on your back, bend the right knee and stretch it across to the left side of the body. Stretch the left arm up over your head. Repeat on the opposite side. This breaks the magnetic field and tunes up the electric field of the body.

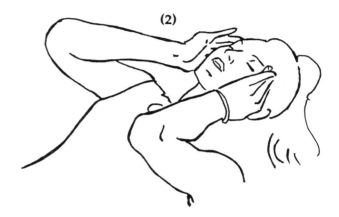

(2)

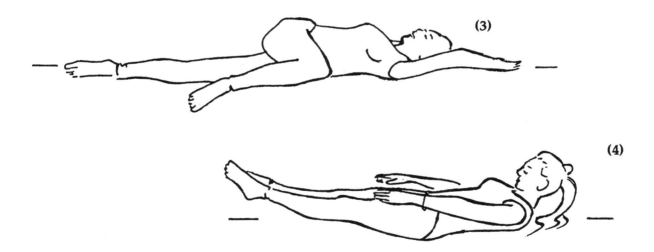

(3)

(4)

4. Do **stretch pose:** Raise the head and feet 6 inches, point the fingers at the toes, and, looking at the feet, begin breath of fire (Chapter 2). Continue for 1-3 min, then inhale, hold the breath in for 15 seconds, exhale and relax (but don't go back to sleep!).

5. Turn onto your right side and pull your knees to your chest for a moment. This strengthens the heart.

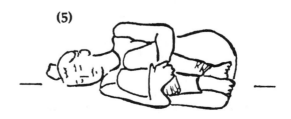

(5)

6. Turn over once more onto your back and pull the knees to the chest with the nose up between the knees, locking the hands around the legs **(a).** Do breath of fire for 1 min, then come into a position sitting on your heels **(b).** Bring the forehead down to the bed for a moment and relax **(c),** breathing normally. This helps eliminate gas from the body.

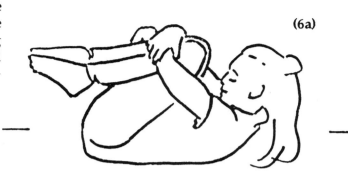

(6a)

(6b)

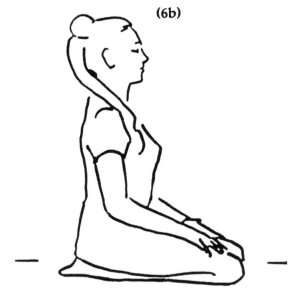

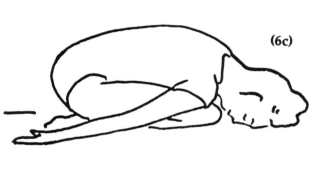

(6c)

7. Lying on the back, rub the palms of the hands and the soles of the feet rapidly together, creating a sensation of heat. This breaks up calcium deposits (crystals) that build up in the hands and feet and allows energy to flow freely through the body.

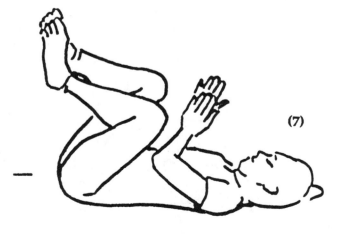

(7)

Getting Up

Remaining barefoot, go into the bathroom. Open and close the cold water tap in the sink a few times to ground the body's electric charge. Using a powder of 1 part salt and 2 parts alum,[3] brush the teeth and gums. Clear the throat. Massage the back of the tongue, gag up mucus, and spit it out as you did before bed. Splash cold water into your open eyes. Massage the body from head to toe with almond oil. (Health food stores carry almond oil as a food item.) Massaging with oil cleanses the pores, and will cut down on the shock of the cold shower you are about to take.

----

[3]Available from some health food stores. Can also be ordered from Harbhajan Singh Khalsa, 2822 Gregory, San Diego, CA 92104 (phone 619-281-1327).

Cold Shower

Next, and most important, take a cold shower. Wear undergarments so that the water does not fall directly on sensitive areas of your body. Step in and out of the water several times, massaging the body vigorously between dunkings. Let the cold water run for a while down your spine and onto the soles of your feet. Cold water is an excellent tonic for the nerves; it improves circulation, destroys mental negativity, and alleviates some kinds of arthritis.[4]

Afterwards, dry off with a rough, coarse towel. Drink two or three glasses of water to help your body flush out toxins accumulated during the night, and you're set for the day!

----

[4]In India, the cold shower is dignified with the title of **Ishnaan,** the science of hydrotherapy. Those who practice this art consider cold water to be "paanee pita," a "fatherly shield" for the body, mind, and soul (see "Ishnaan, the Science of Hydrotherapy" in **Kundalini Yoga for Youth and Joy**).

Appendix B. Kundalini Yoga Teaching Centers

The 3HO Foundation has more than 200 centers offering kundalini yoga instruction as taught by Yogi Bhajan. To find out about the center nearest you, call or write the Regional Center in your area.

Western Region
Hargobind Sadan
2669 Le Conte
Berkeley, CA 94709
(510) 540-6332

Southwestern Region
3HO Foundation Intl Headquarters
House of Guru Ram Das
P.O. Box 351149
Los Angeles, CA 90035
(310) 552-3416

Central Region
Hacienda de Guru Ram Das
Route 3, Box 132D
Espanola, NM 87532
(505) 753-9438

Northwestern Region
Guru Ram Das Ashram
3635 Hilyard Street
Eugene, OR 97405
(503) 686-0432

Southeastern Region
Guru Ram Das Ashram
112 Millbrook Circle
Roswell, GA 30075
(404) 993-6633

Northeastern Region
Guru Ram Das Ashram
368 Village Street
Millis, MA 02054
(508) 376-4525 (3HO)

Midwestern Region
Guru Ram Das Ashram
6036 Marmaduke
St. Louis, MO 63139
(314) 644-3338

Eastern Region
3HO Kundalini Yoga Center
6 Export Drive
Sterling, VA 20164
(703) 430-5551

Canadian Region
The 3HO Kundalini Yoga Center
348 Palmerston Blvd.
Toronto, Ont, Canada M6G 2N6
(416) 929-2507

European Region
3HO Foundation European Headquarters
Den Tex Str 46
Amsterdam, Netherlands 1017 ZC
011-31-20-639-2658

Far Eastern Region
3HO Foundation
Suisha Shinden
Nada-Ku Kobe 657, Japan
011-8178-881-4989

Latin American Region
3HO Foundation
Cacahuatales Coapa
Col. Granjas Coapa Del Tlalpan
Mexico, D.F. Mexico 14330
011-52-56-73-0702

Appendix C. Books on Related Topics

The books in this appendix can be ordered from the following:

[1]Alice B. Clagett, P.O. Box 3142, Santa Monica CA 90408, phone and fax (310) 393-8167. See last pages of **Yoga for Health and Healing** for order form.

[2]Golden Temple Enterprises, Box 13 Shady Lane, Española NM 87532, phone (505) 753-0563, fax (505) 753-5603. Free book, music, and video catalogs available on request.

[3]Ancient Healing Ways, 2545-A Prairie Road, Eugene OR 97402, phone (800) 359-2940 (United States) and (503) 461-2160 x35 (International), fax (503) 461-2191. Free catalog of publications and products for health, healing, and humanity, including audio cassettes and yoga video, available on request.

THE ANCIENT ART OF SELF-HEALING[2,3] by Yogi Bhajan. A veritable encyclopedia of remedies and recommendations for physical and mental health. Prescriptions for almost every part of the body. Includes sections on pregnancy, childbirth, male and female sexual health and hygiene, overweight, underweight, preventive care, and much more. Edited by Dr. Siri Amir Singh Khalsa, D.C.

FOODS FOR HEALTH AND HEALING: REMEDIES AND RECIPES[2,3] based on the teachings of Yogi Bhajan. A popularly priced paperback edition of Yogi Bhajan's teachings on food and health, attractively designed for wide-scale distribution. Based on some of the material in **The Ancient Art of Self-Healing,** this book also contains informative chapters on basic guidelines for healthful eating. There are more than 50 kitchen-tested healing recipes, most of which have never been published before. Buy a copy for yourself and another for a friend or relative.

FROM VEGETABLES, WITH LOVE[2,3] by Siri Ved Kaur Khalsa. An essential collection of gourmet recipes just waiting to come to life in your kitchen. Includes specialties from the Golden Temple restaurants and unique recipes from Yogi Bhajan.

THE GOLDEN TEMPLE VEGETARIAN COOKBOOK[2,3] by Yogi Bhajan. The master of yoga is a master in the kitchen as well. Foods to delight and heal your mind, body, and spirit. Many of the recipes are served at the internationally famous Golden Temple restaurants.

HEALING THROUGH YOGA, MEDITATION, AND MASSAGE[2] by Yogi Bhajan. A course taught by Yogi Bhajan in Barcelona, Spain, on August 16-18, 1985. Includes transcripts of Yogi Bhajan's course, meditations on developing healing energy in the hands, massage techniques, and several yoga sets.

KEEPING UP WITH KUNDALINI YOGA.[2,3] The latest in a series of yoga manuals. Beautifully illustrated. Simple, straightforward instructions. Explanations of the effects of each exercise and a special section devoted to beginners. Sets for elevation, preparation for meditation, metabolism and relaxation, third-eye stimulation, and more.

KUNDALINI YOGA FOR YOUTH AND JOY.[2,3] This manual gives a practical, step-by-step approach for developing a youthful body, an alert mind, and a vibrant projection. Here is a modern method, using time-tested technology, for regenerating and maintaining health, and for dealing with physical stress and mental pressures. Each system of the body is stimulated and balanced.

MAINTENANCE YOGA.[2] A series of rigorous exercise sets designed to stimulate the glandular system and strengthen the nervous system. "Your body is the vehicle of God—a Truth machine. Keep it in tune!" For intermediate students of yoga.

MEDITATION MANUAL. [2,3]A treasury of more than 40 kundalini meditations for the realization of your highest potential. Includes preparatory exercises and explanations of the basic techniques. For intermediate students of yoga.

RELAX AND REJOICE: A MARRIAGE MANUAL[1,2,3] by Yogi Bhajan. How to be joyfully married—and stay that way. Volume 1 contains teachings on love and communication, and special exercises to do with your mate. Volume 2 contains teachings on marriage and sex, including exercises for male potency and a host of meditations for specific marital problems.

SADHANA GUIDELINES.[2,3] Kundalini yoga is the most powerful and effective form of yoga taught today. It is especially suited to the needs of busy people who want to stay calm, bright, and centered in a high-energy world. This book contains complete instructions for your daily practice of this ancient science of awareness, as taught by Yogi Bhajan.

SLIM AND TRIM: EXERCISES AND MEDITATIONS FOR WOMEN.[3] These invigorating yoga sets taught by Yogi Bhajan especially for women are designed for both muscular and structural strength. The meditations build inner strength and security. Together they enhance the total woman.

STRESSAWAY—THE WAY TO RELAX by Gurutej Singh Khalsa and Gordon Briggs. A complete 40-day program for the relief of stress and anxiety through diet, exercise, and keeping still. Beautifully illustrated. *(Note: This book is currently out of print.)*

SURVIVAL KIT—MEDITATIONS AND EXERCISES FOR STRESS AND PRESSURE OF THE TIMES[1,2,3] by Yogi Bhajan. A marvelous collection of meditations for nearly every conceivable emergency, and others to prevent those emergencies from happening. Meditations for atomic radiation, to prepare for earthquake, for insanity, to ward off death, to tranquilize the mind, to alleviate depression, and 25 more. Plus breathing for survival, survival exercises, and exercises and meditations for group consciousness. With clear illustrations and cross indexing.

TRATAKAM MEDITATION PHOTO.[2,3] When you gaze at this specially prepared photo of Yogi Bhajan, your own higher self will speak to you. This 8 by 10 inch photo bears the direct stare of neutrality, an ancient aid to self-guidance. Includes a 4-page article on how to use the photo plus fascinating information on the meditative art of gazing.

YOGA MANUAL.[2,3] A collection of beginners' kundalini yoga exercise and meditation sets with instructions, illustrations, and commentary. An excellent complement to the **Sadhana Guidelines.**

ABOUT YOGI BHAJAN

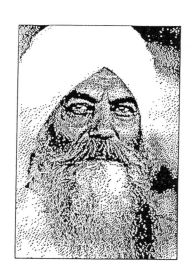

Yogi Bhajan, master of white tantric yoga and kundalini yoga, started teaching in America in January, 1969. He is Director of Spiritual Education for the Healthy, Happy, Holy Organization (3HO), which has expanded to over 100 centers teaching kundalini yoga throughout the world.

Despite the amazing popularity of the spiritual way of life he has inspired in a basically materialistic era, Yoga Bhajan remains a humble and pure channel of the infinite:

"Somebody just shared his knowledge with me, and by the grace of God, I collected it. We are in a desert, and I have a little water with me that I want to share with people. Does that make me a water man? Am I the rain? Am I the clouds? Am I the ocean? No. I am just a little can of water in the desert to which people can touch their lips and think of surviving. Beyond that, I am nothing."

—Yogi Bhajan

Book Order Form

Date: _____

Ordered by:

Name _____

Street _____

City/State/Zip _____

Phone (____) _____

Ship to:

Name _____

Street _____

City/State/Zip _____

Phone (____) _____

Qty.	Name of Book	Item Price	Total Price

Subtotal _____

Shipping and Handling (see chart) _____

Tax (CA only) _____

UPS C.O.D. (add $4.50) _____

GRAND TOTAL _____

Shipping and Handling Charges

Domestic Orders (Continental U.S.)
$0.00 - $19.99.....add $3.95
$20.00 - $49.99.....add $6.95
$50.00 - $99.99.....add $8.95

Hawaii, Alaska, Puerto Rico: Call for shipping quote.
Canada: Add 15%.
International: Prepayment required. Call for shipping quote.
Over $100.00 or Overnight Express: Call for shipping quote.

Please make your check or money order (in U.S. dollars) payable to *Alice B. Clagett*. California residents must pay an 8.25% sales tax. A 40% wholesale discount is available for orders of 10 or more of the same book.

Send your order to:

Alice B. Clagett
P.O. Box 3142, Santa Monica, CA 90408 USA
phone/fax (310) 393-8167